Praise from Lauren Kessler's readers

"I have to thank you for writing such a magnificent book. I read it mornings and evenings on the train, Kleenex in hand, weeping. But laughing, too. I have to thank you for really opening my eyes to the humanity of a group of people I would formerly, out of discomfort and fear, have shunned. You absolutely succeed at revealing the person-ness of your subjects. My (by now very dog-eared) copy will go home to live on the bookshelf dedicated to my fav⁓⁓ ⁓ ks."
—Deborah Way, O ⁓ ⁓ ⁓zine

"I wanted to let you know how i⁓⁓ ⁓aw so much of myself in your pe ⁓ur mother's Alzheimer's. I wish I co ⁓⁓se the way you saw the patients you ⁓⁓ late for that, I will remember her differen⁓⁓
⁓⁓ne Bancroft, California

"Thank you so much for your wonderful book. Both of my grand-mothers had Alzheimer's, along with several aunts. I am seeing signs in my father. Your book gives me a starting place with him that I did not have before. As tragic as the disease is, you gave it a humanity that I did not expect."
—Lynn DeWard, Oregon

"Thank you thank you thank you for such a wonderful book. My fa-ther has Alzheimer's. Your book has helped me immensely, and I now know so much better how to help him."
—Jolynn Ignatovitch, California

"The accounting is riveting, so true—you have captured every mo-ment, every nuance, separated important policy issues from senti-ment and clearly painted painful emotions alongside underlying reason. A Gold Star to you! I have visited over two hundred nursing homes. Daily, my colleagues and I try to make progress in improving our residents' lives. Your book adds depth to both academic long-term care research as well as the field of journalism."
—Karen Reilly, Massachusetts

"I want to sincerely thank you for writing this book. In my opinion, yours is the most realistic portrayal of Alzheimer's ever written. I worked as a nurse's aide in a nursing home back in high school and college. I know all too well how much of our society still wants to avoid thinking about growing older and dying—but your book was superb and very well worth all the time and effort you put into it."
—Sue Ronnenkamp, Texas

PENGUIN BOOKS

FINDING LIFE IN THE LAND OF ALZHEIMER'S

Lauren Kessler is the author of five works of narrative nonfiction, including the *Washington Post* bestseller *Clever Girl* and the *Los Angeles Times* bestseller *The Happy Bottom Riding Club*. Her journalism has appeared in *The New York Times Magazine*; *Los Angeles Times Magazine*; *O, The Oprah Magazine*; and *The Nation*. She directs the graduate program in literary nonfiction at the University of Oregon and lives in Eugene, Oregon.

FINDING LIFE
in the Land of
ALZHEIMER'S

One Daughter's Hopeful Story

LAUREN KESSLER

PENGUIN BOOKS

Previously published as *Dancing with Rose*

PENGUIN BOOKS

Published by the Penguin Group

Penguin Group (USA) Inc., 375 Hudson Street, New York, New York 10014, U.S.A.

Penguin Group (Canada), 90 Eglinton Avenue East, Suite 700, Toronto,
Ontario, Canada M4P 2Y3 (a division of Pearson Penguin Canada Inc.)

Penguin Books Ltd, 80 Strand, London WC2R 0RL, England

Penguin Ireland, 25 St Stephen's Green, Dublin 2, Ireland
(a division of Penguin Books Ltd)

Penguin Group (Australia), 250 Camberwell Road, Camberwell,
Victoria 3124, Australia (a division of Pearson Australia Group Pty Ltd)

Penguin Books India Pvt Ltd, 11 Community Centre,
Panchsheel Park, New Delhi – 110 017, India

Penguin Group (NZ), 67 Apollo Drive, Rosedale, North Shore 0632,
New Zealand (a division of Pearson New Zealand Ltd)

Penguin Books (South Africa) (Pty) Ltd, 24 Sturdee Avenue,
Rosebank, Johannesburg 2196, South Africa

Penguin Books Ltd, Registered Offices:
80 Strand, London WC2R 0RL, England

First published in the United States of America as *Dancing with Rose* by
Viking Penguin, a member of Penguin Group (USA) Inc. 2007
Published in Penguin Books 2008

1 3 5 7 9 10 8 6 4 2

THE LIBRARY OF CONGRESS HAS CATALOGED THE HARDCOVER EDITION AS FOLLOWS:
Kessler, Lauren.
Dancing with Rose : finding life in the land of Alzheimer's / Lauren Kessler.
p. cm.
ISBN 978-0-670-03859-6 (hc.)
ISBN 978-0-14-311368-3 (pbk.)
1. Kessler, Lauren. 2. Alzheimer's disease—Patients—Care.
3. Caregivers. I. Title.
RC523K47   2007
362.196'831—dc22   2006035699

Printed in the United States of America
Designed by Carla Bolte • Set in ITC Garamond Light

for
Marguerite Lillian
and
Sidney NMI

This is the true wine of
astonishment:

We are not
Over
When we think
We are.

—Alice Walker

Author's Note

This is a work of nonfiction. Maplewood is a real place, but that is not its real name. The people in this book—the residents of Maplewood, their families, the institutional caregivers, and the administrators—are real people. I've changed some of the names to ensure privacy, but in only one small instance (a hometown) have I knowingly changed any facts or details about their lives. The events and incidents chronicled in the book happened. Those few I did not directly witness I reconstructed based on interviews with those who were present. All of the conversations recorded in the book took place. I heard them (and participated in many of them) and wrote them down in my reporter's notebook at the time or soon thereafter.

Any liberties I have taken are liberties not of fact but of interpretation. I saw this place, these people, these events through my own eyes and filtered them, as all nonfiction writers do, through my own sensibilities. I mean to tell truths both factual and emotional.

1

To apply for this entry-level, minimum-wage job I have to fill out thirty-two pages of forms, including a Criminal History Request, a Substance Abuse Control and Management Policy form, a Nondiscrimination and Harassment Policy Statement, a Workplace Violence Statement (no weapons, no stalking, no "hostile behavior"), a Department of Justice Employment Eligibility Verification form, a Tuberculin Screening Program form, a hepatitis B vaccine form, two IRS forms, an Employee Input Worksheet and, oh yes, a job application. I also have to pee in a jar, assuring my future employers that on this day, August 5, 2004, I did not have cocaine, methamphetamine, morphine, PCP, or THC in my system. On the application there is no space to list my advanced degrees—and no reason to list them. I don't need even a high school diploma to qualify for this job.

There is, however, a space for "special skills." I think hard about this: Archival research? Pilates? Italian cooking? I don't think that's what they mean. But surely there is something I know how to do that qualifies me for this job as an RA (Resident

Assistant) at Maplewood. Maplewood is a place for people with Alzheimer's; its RAs are the unskilled, hands-on caregivers who do all the dirty work. I could put down that my mother had Alzheimer's, but I'm afraid that my special skill there was denial. I did feed her sometimes when I visited the care facility she lived in near the end of her life, and sometimes I brushed her teeth. I write down "personal care" in the space provided.

It doesn't really matter. I have the job regardless of what I write on the application. I am just going through the motions to make it official. I've worked it all out with the administrator of the facility. She knows me, as does the entire staff, because I have been visiting this place on and off for months, observing the women and men who live here. I was working on a magazine story, and I was, I thought, working on myself. Eight years ago I had faced my mother's illness and my mother's death with a combination of fear and detachment, with emotions shut down and, I felt, lessons unlearned. Although I had managed not to learn much, I knew I *should* have learned something, that the higher function of a big, awful event like this is supposed to be at least instructive if not life altering. And so, writer that I was, I had decided to write about Alzheimer's. I was going to force myself to confront what I'd been too scared to confront earlier, when the disease had been up close and personal. I was going to buckle down and learn all manner of important life lessons. I was going to make up for being a lousy daughter. This Alzheimer's magazine story was to be redemptive.

So I spent time in the trenches observing other people's mothers, and I wrote about it. I peeled away maybe a layer or two, but I didn't feel much wiser. I had reached an impasse, and I thought I knew why. It was the distance I was keeping, the shield I was holding in front of myself to deflect the really tough stuff. It was my detached position as observer and writer. If I was to come to terms with this disease that took my mother's life, if I was to learn whatever it was I needed to learn, I had to stop hiding behind my reporter's notebook and get inside the world of Alzheimer's. And so, with the knowledge and permission of the staff—this was no undercover operation—I decided to hire on at Maplewood. I would immerse myself fully and completely in the daily lives of those with this disease. I would take care of other people's mothers the way strangers had taken care of my mother.

I thought I knew what I was facing. I had read the medical reports, with their chronicles of unstoppable brain plaques, impenetrable neural tangles, and shrunken cerebral cortexes. I had read the heart-wrenching stories in the media, seen the documentaries. I had experienced my own mother's demise, her five-year transformation from the dotty aunt who makes you laugh at the occasional inappropriate remark to the old woman who can no longer feed herself. This was a disease that fractured life, that erased the past, that scoured the body of its remembered self. The portrait of Alzheimer's I had in my head was unremittingly bleak. I figured I could stand the job for maybe two weeks.

There are five of us waiting in the lobby of Maplewood at 8:20 the next morning: three women in their early twenties, a thin, sandy-haired young man who looks as if he doesn't need to shave every day, and me. Christine, who worked her way up from RA (Resident Assistant, the bottom-rung job I'm here for) to MA (Medication Aide, the shift supervisor empowered to dispense meds) to her current position of Resident Care Coordinator, is running the show. She's a tough-looking woman, hard worked, her hair brittle from home perms, her smile weary. She's twenty-eight. When Christine comes out to the lobby, she doesn't welcome us or introduce herself or offer a summary of what we can expect for the next six hours. Instead, she takes us back to the closet-sized, windowless break room, shows us a tiny refrigerator and a vending machine stocked with junk food, and tells us to clock in. We learn, before anything else, that we have a three-minute leeway when we clock in for our shift. If we punch in any later than 6:33 in the morning, we're considered late. Three late days, we are told, is grounds for termination. We also learn that if we are ill, we have to find our own replacement. If we can't, we must come in to work. If we don't come to work, we're fired. I'm more astonished than I should be.

This is the way the world of minimum-wage work operates. I've always worked for a living, but except for the usual scut jobs that saw me through college, I've led the sheltered, benefit-buffered life of a middle-class professional. After the sobering mini-lecture about all the reasons we could get fired, we are led back to the meeting room in the atrium at the center of the facility, where two-inch-thick packets of material await us. Christine tells us that we will start with the first document in the packet, the Employee Orientation Manual, which we will read aloud, each of us reading a page.

This is what we're going to do for the next five hours and fifty-four minutes? I can't believe it. I can read this stuff at home. But, as I listen to the sometimes halting recitation of my fellow trainees, as I hear one struggle to pronounce the word *collaboration* and another stumble over the word *Alzheimer's,* I realize that Christine is right to have us read aloud. Two of my three fellow trainees could not possibly read this material themselves without help.

In one of the several dozen documents we read, the responsibilities of the RA position are summarized as "performing care with an awareness of dignity and individuality." I like the pleasing, high-minded language (and the thought behind it), but I know from my own observations that it obscures the unpleasant daily details of the job: toileting, changing diapers, emptying commodes, showering, dressing and undressing, serving food, hand-feeding, doing laundry, vacuuming, dusting, disinfecting, taking out the garbage. There are other duties as well: getting people to and from scheduled activities, keeping a detailed written log of whatever happens on your shift, dealing with relatives who come to visit, and, maybe most important, just simply *being there* for the people for whom Maplewood is home, speaking softly, reassuringly, answering the same question two dozen times. I am exhausted just thinking about it. Like all mothers, I have done these jobs, *all* of these jobs. But caring for children who are cute and cuddly and smell good and get smarter every day is just not the same.

Eight years ago I cared for my mother on my own for exactly eighteen hours—I consulted my watch often—beginning when my husband and I picked her up at the airport (I paid for a geriatric nurse to accompany her on the cross-country flight from New York) and ending when I signed her in at the care facility the next afternoon. I was terrified the entire time, from the ride in the backseat, where I tried to chat with a woman who looked somewhat like my mother but couldn't be my mother because she had no idea who I was—me, her firstborn, her only daughter, her bête noire—to the moment I hugged her good-bye in the room I carefully decorated with things she no longer recognized as her own.

It was early evening when we drove out to the airport to get her. My father had been caring for her back in New York for several years by then. She had deteriorated from pleasantly addled, a stage my father refused to acknowledge because to him my mother had *always* been addled, to the can't-drive-a-car stage (she had gotten into a fender bender and had driven away, oblivious, before my father yanked her license) to the wet-the-bed, wander-the-neighborhood phase. He was doing the best he could for a guy who had so little patience with illness that he used to glare at me across the dinner table when I sneezed. He thought I got sick on purpose just to annoy him. But my father had, in fact, stepped up in a big way. He was in his early seventies then and not a bad-looking guy. He had a full head of hair. He played a respectable game of tennis. He had a great government pension. He was, in other words, a "catch." He could have stashed my mother somewhere and found himself a girlfriend—more likely, she would have found him—and had some fun. He didn't. He learned how to run the house, how to do the grocery shopping, how to cook and clean. He did it all himself—I hadn't come home once to help, and my brother had his own life in Florida—and he had settled in for the long haul.

I was astonished. I didn't think he loved her enough to do what he was doing. I didn't think he loved her at all. My parents had not enjoyed a happy marriage. I grew up pretending not to notice how ugly it got sometimes, not ugly like wife-battering ugly or throwing-the-crockery ugly or write-a-memoir-about-it ugly, but subtler and more sinister: hissing fights behind closed doors; withering looks across the dinner table, my father muttering under his breath, every night, about my mother's faults, just loud enough for everyone to hear; my mother wincing, retreating, creating distance, growing colder. I grew up secretly hoping they'd divorce, and I could go live with my mother who'd get a job as a clothes designer in Manhattan, and we'd stay up late every night watching Katharine Hepburn movies on channel 9 and eating brussels sprouts, which my father hated. I grew up plotting my escape. My father was the villain in this domestic drama, my mother the creative spirit squelched by an emotional bully. For years, for decades, for my whole life, he had been the bad guy. Now, all of a sudden, he was the good guy. It didn't come easy, but I had to admire him.

But after four years of caring for my mother, he was exhausted, and his own health was beginning to suffer. He needed a break. Three thousand miles away, I needed to feel like I was doing something in the midst of this family tragedy. I had made good my escape after high school and pretty much disappeared from the family after college, an estranged daughter who wanted no part of her own past. But so much water had gone under that bridge that the river, the very contours of the river, had long changed. I was a mother now—three times over—and I knew something about the parent-child bond from the other side. Maybe I owed both of them more than I thought, more than I had wanted to admit. At any rate, I knew it was my turn. And so, a continent away from my parents, I talked to the people at the local Alzheimer's Association office, consulted with geriatricians, interviewed eldercare specialists, and visited care facilities in my town. Then I persuaded my father to send my mother West, where she would be cared for in what I had concluded was the best Alzheimer's facility in town.

Getting off the plane, she looked a little better than I expected—I hadn't seen her in almost ten years—her hair freshly colored and coiffed, her navy pantsuit AARP acceptable, her eyes clear and focused, a faded blue, like jeans that have been through too many washes. She was pleasant and well mannered, treating my husband and me like marginally interesting strangers. She didn't object to getting in the car with us. She asked no questions about where she was going or who we were. I, of course, did all the wrong things, quizzing her endlessly in the backseat: "You remember who I am, don't you, Mom? Lauren, remember me, Lauren, your daughter? And this is Tom, remember Tom? We're married. You came to our wedding, remember?" I don't know how many times I said the word *remember* to this woman who had a brain disease that robbed her of her memory.

When we got home, it was clear that she was tired. She had traveled across three time zones and was ready for bed. I was thankful because I had no idea what I was going to do with her otherwise. I showed her the guest room I had prepared. There was a thick featherbed on top of the mattress and a down comforter over it. It looked like a puffy cloud. My mother would have loved it. She had an artist's eye for beauty—she was, she had been, a talented amateur painter of still lifes—and she, like me, had a penchant for high-thread-count bed linen. But this woman didn't notice. I opened her suitcase and looked for a nightgown. All her nightgowns were flimsy, sleeveless polyester things, cold and slimy to the touch. I went upstairs and got one of my long-sleeved flannel gowns and put it on her bed. I wasn't sure what she could do, what I was supposed to do. I told her it was time for bed, that she should get herself ready, and I left her there. Ten minutes later she was still sitting on the bed dressed in her traveling clothes. I started to undress her—no big deal—until I came to the diaper. I had forgotten she was in diapers.

With two sons and a daughter, I had changed a lot of diapers. In fact, when my mother arrived in town that fall, my daughter was only a few months old, and I was a good two years away from the end of my diaper-changing days. But changing your child's diaper is entirely different from changing your mother's. The first is a minor chore; the second, a heartbreak. I cleaned her up, then dressed her in my nightgown, led her to bed, and tucked her in. She smelled sour, vinegary, this woman who never used to leave the house without dabbing Crêpe de Chine behind her ears.

"I won't be able to sleep," she told me. I pulled a chair next to the bed and sat down. I thought about holding her hand. Or rather, I thought about what a nice scene that would make, me holding her hand. I thought about how that's what a good, loving daughter would do. She was asleep in five minutes.

When I woke the next morning, I rushed downstairs to see how she was and panicked when I saw the bed was empty. She got out of the house, I thought. She's wandering somewhere. She's going to be run over by a car, and it will be my fault. *My father will kill me.* But my mother had not escaped. She was in the kitchen eating a piece of toast she had made for herself, miraculously locating bread, toaster, butter, knife, and plate in a house she'd never before visited. My mother's domain had been the kitchen, and not just in the prosaic sense of a suburban housewife of the '50s and '60s. My mother had been an enthusiastic and inventive cook, an early Julia Child acolyte, a woman who taught herself Chinese cooking and periodically took the Long Island Rail Road into the city to buy exotic spices and sauces in Chinatown. This was decades before you could find such items on the "ethnic food" aisle at the A&P, decades before any suburban housewife even *knew* there were such items. Kitchen knowledge, it seemed, knowledge of anyone's kitchen, was hardwired.

A few hours later, I dropped off my mother at the care facility (not Maplewood, which was yet to be built), a clean, modern, trying-hard-not-to-be-institutional place with six vacant-eyed women sitting in the living room. I got out of there as fast as I could. When I got home I took the nightgown she had worn, the one I lent her, and put it in the trash. Just in case Alzheimer's was contagious.

That is the sum of my experience caring for a person with Alzheimer's. I am as unqualified for this RA job as a person can be, perhaps more unqualified than someone who's never had to confront the disease before, who doesn't have a wellspring of fear and loathing. The responsibilities unhinge me. Suppose someone in my care slips and falls? Suppose someone has a reaction to a medication? Suppose someone chokes on her food? Suppose I—overeducated, overachiever that I am, a person who can make just about anything into a contest and is never happy with second place—suppose I can't do this job?

But what I am most scared of is reencountering the disease this intimately. I know I still have so much left to, as they say, "process" about my mother's illness, about my own fears of growing old, of getting sick, of being dependent, of dying. I need to do this. I think we all need to do this. It has something to do growing into the second half of your life. For me, it has something to do with making posthumous peace with my mother. And, I must admit, it has something to do with racking up badly needed karma points. As a daughter I am deep into negative territory.

At the end of the orientation session, I finish all the paperwork and hand it to Brooke, Maplewood's administrator and my soon-to-be boss. She is a tall, willowy young woman in her midtwenties, with creamy skin and immense brown eyes. She is full of indiscriminate girlish enthusiasm about everything, from the cold pork chop she will eat for lunch to the new flower pots that hang over the entrance to Maplewood. She has been enthusiastic about my presence since I started observing months ago. She believes she does good work, and, like so many who work at Maplewood, she loves what she does. To her, this is not a place of tragedy and despair—despite the tragic and despairing public face Alzheimer's has. It is rather a vibrant community of quirky souls. It is her job to keep the community together, to keep it functioning, and, beyond that, to keep it *fun*—which is not a word that would occur to most people when describing Alzheimer's care.

Brooke walks out of her small office waving my paperwork over her head and announcing loudly, for any nearby staff to hear, "Look, we just hired Lauren!" Patty, the woman who sits at the front desk and with whom I have had two or three entirely casual encounters, comes running over. She gives me a full-body hug that leaves me breathless.

2

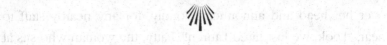

Maplewood is part of a sprawling eldercare community that sits on a vast tract of former orchard land north of town. Around the perimeter of the ten-acre site are small cottages inhabited by active retirees. In the center is an expansive, two-story assisted-living facility for those who can no longer live independently. Across a manicured lawn and two parking lots sits Maplewood, designed specifically to care for those with Alzheimer's. A person could spend the last two or three decades of life on this campus, entering as a cottage-dweller, graduating to assisted living when the time came and then, in the unlucky event of dementia, transferring to Maplewood. This continuity of care concept, also known as "aging in place," is the current ne plus ultra of the booming eldercare industry. This community was built less than five years ago.

From the outside, Maplewood looks like a well-maintained, moderately priced motel, maybe a Comfort Inn, with that stolid, inoffensive style of architecture that is without region or personality. Inside it is clean, bright, modern, and not nearly as institutional as one might expect. The walls of the lobby are lined with mahogany-stained bookcases. The large, square indoor atrium that forms the core of the facility is landscaped with real trees, dotted with park benches and a wooden gazebo, and populated by happily chirping birds in outsized cages. Through double doors at the corners of the atrium are four self-contained residential units known as "neighborhoods." In each neighborhood, fourteen single rooms, most with attached private baths, surround a large, sky-lit common area that functions as living room, kitchen, dining room, and den. In each neighborhood, a door leads from the common area to a pleasantly landscaped outdoor patio and garden.

The place is state-of-the-art, part of the recent revolution in the design of environments for those with Alzheimer's. A bonafide epidemic now, with an estimated 4.5 million people affected by the disease, perhaps a third of whom are housed in "memory care" facilities, Alzheimer's has attracted its own subset of architects and interior designers. The neighborhood concept embraced by Maplewood scales down the world while leaving its essentials intact. The small, homey, open settings, unlike the long corridors of old-fashioned nursing homes, are designed to feel both familiar and negotiable. The skylights in the common area, along with recessed lighting and plenty of lamps, eliminate shadows, which are thought to be particularly frightening to those with Alzheimer's. The doors that connect the neighborhoods to the atrium are always open, and the doors to the outdoor patios are never locked. This design recognizes and allows for one of the hallmark behaviors of Alzheimer's—wandering. There is no way for a resident to "escape" this place—the outdoor patios are fully enclosed, the doors from the atrium to the outside world are locked and key-coded—yet the open design gives a feeling of freedom.

On the first day of training I find myself in neighborhood 3 along with a fellow trainee named Jasmine. Frances, a moon-faced, soft-spoken, utterly calm young woman from Guam, is our trainer. She is one of the old-timers at Maplewood, having been employed here for eight months. Most Resident Assistants don't last long, Frances says matter-of-factly. The job is too tough. The pay is too low. The benefits are skimpy, and a long time coming. You have to work full-time for three months to qualify for any health benefits here, and few RAs stay at Maplewood—or any eldercare facility—for that long. A lot of money was invested in building this place, but not a lot is spent on the staff who keep it going. The RAs and the kitchen staff work for minimum wage with negligible raises awarded after lengthy service. The Med Aides, the next step up in the hierarchy, make maybe twenty-five cents an hour more. The facility administrator, one of the few salaried employees and the only one except for the nurse who needs a college degree to qualify for the job, earns the equivalent of eleven or twelve dollars an hour if you account for all the overtime and weekend work. The turnover is high, from top to bottom.

Frances is not complaining, and she's not trying to discourage us. She's just getting a little weary of training new workers, some who don't make it past the three-day orientation, others who stay only long enough to pick up their first paycheck. Frances understands why others come and go. She accepts the reality. But it's not her reality. She loves this job, she tells us. She is one of those earnest, hardworking, egoless people you read about but don't quite believe exist. She comes from an extended close-knit family of recent immigrants, has a four-year-old son at home, and works full-time while taking night classes at the local community college. Someday she'd like to be an RN.

Jasmine, my fellow trainee, is a big girl, almost six feet tall, solidly built, with thick dyed-black hair and a lot of missing teeth. Most of her molars have been pulled because, she tells me, shrugging her shoulders, she never had money to go to the dentist, and none of her jobs ever provided dental insurance. She was sixteen when she got pregnant and seventeen when she had her son. She's twenty-four now and has been with a series of loser men and worked at a series of loser jobs. Her last job was at Target unloading trucks. She had to report for work at 3:30 in the morning, which meant awakening her son at 2:30 and carting him who-knows-where for childcare. Jasmine and I have as little in common as two female humans can have, yet this morning we bond almost instantly over our shared insecurities and our collective panic about this job neither of us thinks she can do.

For the next three days, Jasmine and I will be training in this neighborhood, currently home to eleven Alzheimer's patients. At Maplewood, the population ranges from high-functioning folks who are communicative and can take reasonable care of some of their personal needs to frail, silent, wheelchair-bound people who require complete assistance with all daily activities. Although these higher-functioning folks are the healthiest people here, they are not at the beginning stages of Alzheimer's. At that stage—the mild memory loss, slight confusion, something's-not-quite-right stage—people often cover up the symptoms or learn to compensate, and those around them either fail or refuse to see the signs. By the time people reach a place like Maplewood, the disease has progressed to a point where their care is not only beyond their own capabilities but also beyond their families'. It could be something simple: a 180-pound man can no longer get himself undressed, into the shower, and bathed, and his 120-pound wife will hurt herself, and maybe him, trying. Or a woman whose husband is no longer alive and whose children live thousands of miles away and have children and complicated lives of their own can no longer drive to the store to buy groceries. Or a person with the most loving, selfless, involved family progresses to a point where twenty-four-hour supervision is necessary, and the family just can't do it. The myth is that families dump their relatives in institutions like Maplewood. The reality is that the decision is an agonizing one frequently made after extraordinary, often long-term, efforts to care for the person at home.

The road to a place like Maplewood, or the facility I found for my mother, is a long one that begins with that first tiny hint, the hint you try to ignore or explain away, that something might be wrong. Years before she got into that fender bender and drove away, I knew something was not right with my mother. It wasn't failing memory as much as it was off-kilter behavior: a flash of anger that seemed to come from nowhere, inattention, fogginess, a kind of disconnect, as if ordinary life sometimes didn't quite make sense to her. I remember the exact moment I admitted to myself that something was wrong. My mother was visiting. I came home from work and found her down in the basement ironing her way through a pile of my husband's dirty shirts. When I told her the clothes hadn't been washed yet, she smiled at me absently, nodded, and kept ironing.

I thought she was going deaf. I thought she was drinking. I never thought Alzheimer's. She came from a long line of long-lived females: her mother, then a spunky ninety, was quick-witted, funny, and upbeat. Her grandmother had lived into her late eighties. Her great-grandmother, whom the family called Old Oldie, had lived, all faculties intact, to 102.

While I was noticing—and making excuses for—the changes in my mother's behavior, real physiological changes were happening inside her brain. Scientists don't know yet what causes Alzheimer's, but they are at least beginning to unravel the sequence of neurological events that results in the disease. Inside my mother's brain was a gluey substance that was slowly, inexorably, mucking up the works by creating clumps of plaque, like the kind inside clogged arteries, tangled bundles and maybe, according to the most recent research, rodlike aggregates that got in the way of the nerve impulses that made the brain work. At first it was thought that this gluey substance (beta amyloid protein is its name) was invading from another part of the body. But researchers now believe the protein is part of normal brain chemistry and that it actually has an important function. The problem was my mother's gluey protein got out of hand because of a breakdown in an internal regulation system. Scientists think there are other cells in the brain, janitor cells, whose job it is to clean up excess gluey protein. In a normal brain, the janitors are diligent. In the Alzheimer's brain, in my mother's brain, the janitors were not.

Why does that happen? Why did it happen to *my* mother? This is part of the stubborn, ongoing mystery of the disease. You can read the research in reverse for hints—I certainly have— looking at the studies that parse out who is less likely to get Alzheimer's: people who exercise, people who get regular mental stimulation, people who have an active social life, people who drink only in moderation, who don't smoke, who don't eat red meat. Each one of these behaviors is in some way linked to a healthy brain. Does that mean that the opposite behaviors help cause the disease? Maybe. If so, in retrospect, my mother was a poster girl for bad behavior, and the disease was a foregone conclusion. She smoked, she drank, she ate red meat. She didn't exercise. For most of the last twenty years of her life, she did little that was mentally stimulating. She was socially isolated, depressed. Did all of these factors, or any of them, or a certain combination somehow cause the chemical imbalance in her brain? Medical science has yet to figure this out.

My mother's decline, however it happened, happened in stages. There's one particularly compelling theory about the progress of the disease. It explains the decline in function as a regression through four successively earlier periods of life. In early stage Alzheimer's, the theory goes, adult learning is lost. The person forgets the most recently acquired skills like driving a car or writing a check. There are some problems finding just the right word, a decreasing interest in the world, some indifference to the normal courtesies of adult life. In what's called early-mid phase, adolescent learning is lost. Retention and recall suffers. Normal routines are forgotten. The person may become angry or hostile—like a teenager—with frequent outbursts, which are known in Alzheimer's circles as "incontinence of emotion." In late-mid phase, childhood learning is lost. The person becomes disoriented to time and place and people. Language reverts to simple words or repetition. Modesty disappears. In the late-terminal phase, infancy learning is lost, and the person, like a baby, is incapable of caring for herself. She is incontinent, unable to dress, bathe, or feed herself. She has lost language and has little response to stimuli. She begins to lose weight. This final decline is termed "failure to thrive," the same terminology used for ailing infants.

It's interesting, and maybe in an odd way comforting, to think of the disease this way—orderly, understandable, predictable. But the truth is, Alzheimer's manifests itself differently in every person and progresses at very different speeds. When I spent time with my mother at the facility I chose for her, I saw women who sat motionless and stared out into space for hours, women who couldn't keep still, women who never spoke, and women who never shut up. I saw two women, both the same age, who had been diagnosed the same year, one of whom was catatonic, the other of whom read the newspaper every day. Watching my mother, I came to my own unofficial staging of the disease.

Stage I: I forgot what I bought at the store for dinner.

Stage II: I forgot how to cook dinner.

Stage III: I forgot how to eat dinner.

Some of the Alzheimer's patients in this Maplewood neighborhood are, according to what Frances tells me and Jasmine, in my unofficial stage II category; others have devolved to stage III. As I ask about them, Frances cautions me—just as Christine emphasized in yesterday's orientation—that we are not to call them "patients." We refer to them as "residents," which makes sense. Maplewood is not a hospital or a skilled nursing facility. It is a home. These people live here. Most will live here until they die.

Today training means watching Frances, asking questions, and attempting some of the lighter tasks. Frances tells us that the first thing we do when we come in is check the "comm log," a black binder stored in a cabinet under the counter in the kitchenette. In the comm log we'll find the "S/L schedule" (who gets a shower this morning, whose laundry we are to do today), the dietary chart (who gets regular meals, and who gets "extra portion," "no fish," "no eggs," "cut-up only," "puree only"), and notes scribbled by the swing- and night-shift caregivers: "131 0% bkfst," "138 refused shower," "141 out for lunch w/ daughter," "136 up all nite." We are supposed to refer to the residents by room number, not name—not to their faces, of course, but in all paperwork and to each other when we talk on the walkie-talkies clipped to our half-aprons.

I'm amazed to learn this. This is a place intent on being homey. Among our duties, Frances tells us, is baking cookies every afternoon, so that the neighborhoods always smell like grandma's kitchen. Using numbers, not names, seems a particularly dehumanizing thing to do. Frances says it's some kind of privacy issue, but, whatever the rationale, it immediately complicates the job. I will have to memorize not only names but the room numbers that match.

It's 6:45 a.m., just fifteen minutes into our first day of training, and Jasmine and I are quietly freaking out. We exchange deer-in-the-headlights glances whenever Frances isn't looking. We have to wake up eleven people, two of whom, the frailest, we will have to heft out of bed and into wheelchairs by looping a wide canvas belt around their middles and grabbing back and front. This is a two-person operation, or as Frances calls it, a "two-person assist." Three of the eleven residents can still pretty much take care of themselves, but for the others we undress them, clean up those in adult diapers who were incontinent during the night, sit them on the toilet and coax them to use it, clean them again, pick out their clothes and dress them, brush their teeth (or dentures), comb their hair, shave the men, and get them all out to the dining area for breakfast by 8:15. Two of these people also require showers in the morning, as per the rotating S/L schedule. Most of the residents need our full assistance in the shower, including washing all parts of their bodies.

Frances tells us what we already noted in the comm log—that some residents are very difficult to coax into the shower, flatly refusing and becoming agitated if the point is pressed. It's not uncommon for people with Alzheimer's to dislike bathing. No one really knows why, but one idea I've heard is that it has to do with skin sensitivity. It's not because their aging skin is thin and fragile, which is true, but, so this theory goes, because as their other senses have dulled, their sense of touch has sharpened. And so temperature changes, pressure, the rubbing of clothes are all felt with a new—and uncomfortable—intensity. Frances says that if a resident refuses a shower we have to try three different strategies, which I guess we make up on the fly, record exactly what we tried on the official Shower Refusal Form, sign and date it, and give it to the next in command.

Frances talks to us as she works, explaining the duties and detailing the level of care needed for each resident as she puts on the first of what will be this morning's fifteen sets of latex gloves. She is using multiple wipes to clean the rear of 131 (whose name happens also to be Frances), who has had a moderately sloppy BM either between 6:00 a.m., when the night shift caregiver was supposed to do the final check, and 6:45, when Frances checked, or, more likely, sometime during the night. The night staff—here called "noc" for nocturnal rather than the ominous and more common term "graveyard"—is rumored to be a bunch of slackers who choose to work the unhours (10:30 p.m. to 6:30 a.m.) because no one in administration is around to look over their shoulders, and no families are likely to visit and see what goes on.

Next we knock on 140's (Marianne's) door to tell her it's time to get up. She is, Frances says, the easiest person to care for in the neighborhood. She dresses herself (impeccably) and takes care of all her own hygiene and personal care. Marianne turns out to be a pleasant, competent, articulate woman who looks just like what she is—a retired university administrator—and not at all like what she has become—a victim of Alzheimer's. I ask Frances why Marianne is here. She seems entirely capable of taking care of herself. She seems, well, *normal.* Frances smiles. "You'll see," she says.

Then it's on to 141, where we find Eloise, a gracious woman who awakens with a smile and thanks the three of us for coming in to help her. We pick out her clothes, which speak to both her social class (silk blouses, decent costume jewelry) and the attentiveness of her family (no missing buttons, no stretched-out waistbands). Then we walk her into the bathroom, slip off her nightgown, pull down her diaper, sit her on the toilet and start dressing her while she pees. Eloise has very bad edema—one of her ankles is twice the size of the other—and needs to wear thick thigh-high compression stockings that are incredibly difficult to get on. She brushes her own teeth. Frances applies lipstick.

Our next stop is room 129, home to, oh my God, *another* Frances. That means two residents living two doors apart are named Frances, plus the woman who is training us. Could this be any harder? This Frances, Frances M., has woken up in the middle of the night and peed all over her carpet. When we open the door to her room, the air is hot and so pungent it stings our nostrils. I go to fling open the windows but find that they self-lock at six inches. Frances, our trainer, sends me to the utility closet to get a bottle of super-disinfectant spray called "Shock." We'll spray the rug when Frances M. is out of the room and call Jim the janitor to shampoo it later today.

An hour into the morning, and I'm sweating through my cheap polyester uniform shirt (an unbecoming dusky maroon), wondering why exactly I'm doing this. Perhaps I don't really need to make posthumous peace with my mother. And there must be easier ways to rack up good karma. Can the job really be as hard as it appears? How do all these women—just about all the caregivers here are women—do it? And why? You can make two dollars an hour more as a grocery store checker, where, standing upright and in comfort, you can banter with pleasant shoppers while you *scan* packages of Depends rather than *use* the product (and all that entails) on real people. It's been twenty years since I've confronted a work situation that I could not handle with ease.

By 8:20 all eleven residents are sitting at three tables, placemats and silverware set before each, glasses of water or juice or both, cups of coffee for those who want it. Hayes, who is ninety-one, is currently the only man in the neighborhood. In the world of Alzheimer's, as in the larger word of the elderly, women significantly outnumber men. At Maplewood right now, of thirty-nine residents living in four neighborhoods, only four are men. Hayes is the oldest and has been here the longest.

Hayes's wife of sixty-eight years, Mabel, has specified exactly how he is to be dressed every morning: white cotton undershirt, long-sleeved button-down sport shirt, V-neck sweater on top; underwear, long johns, and khakis on bottom. He is unable to help much, so it takes forever to dress him. But I must admit, the guy looks dapper. He is tall and just barely on the scrawny side of lean with a chiseled face, a strong jaw, and a becoming wisp of silver hair. If Jeremy Irons lives to be a nonagenarian, he'll look just like Hayes.

Frances, Jasmine, and I are sorting through the covered breakfast plates on the cart that was just brought in, checking the dietary log to make sure we give each resident what the log says we should give them. Somehow Frances has this memorized: no eggs for 135, she tells us; cut-ups to 131, finger food for 134. She says this faster than I can find the notations in the book. Jasmine and I exchange another look while Frances's back is turned. The look is equal parts awe and terror. This isn't even Frances's regularly assigned neighborhood. She usually works neighborhood 1. But apparently she's worked relief here enough to know everything there is to know. I want to admire her competence, but instead I am intimidated. I'd dislike her if she weren't so likable.

Meanwhile, from over at one of the small dining room tables, Hayes starts yelling.

"Help me, help me, somebody help me!"

We all look over at the same time to make sure nothing is wrong. Hayes is sitting up straight in his wheelchair. He's got a glass of milk in his hand.

"Help me, help me!" he yells again. As Frances and Jasmine hand out the plates, I go over to see what's up with Hayes. He doesn't seem to need help, and when I ask him what he needs, he doesn't know. I stand next to him and rub his back, the only thing I can think to do. That quiets him down. When I leave a minute later to get his plate, he starts yelling again. I hurry back.

"I'm Hayes," Hayes says when I walk up to him.

"Hello," I say. "I'm Lauren." He looks up at me.

"Moron?" he says.

"No," I say, taken aback for a moment, then laughing. "LAW-REN," I say my name loud and clear, articulating the syllables carefully.

"MORE-ON?" he says again, also articulating, also loud and clear.

Is he doing this on purpose? I start to say my name again but think better of it.

"How do you do, Hayes?" I ask.

"I do as I please," he replies.

I laugh so hard that Frances comes over to see if I'm okay. Who knew that an Alzheimer's patient—I mean *resident*—could deliver lines like a Borscht Belt comedian? I'm going to like this Hayes, even if he is a handful.

"Rub my back," he orders me. "I'm itchy. I'm itchy."

The plates are distributed, more coffee (decaf, of course) is

poured, and plastic juice glasses are refilled. Frances feeds one
of the Franceses—the almost centenarian whom I decide to call
"Old Frances" from now on—and Jasmine feeds Addie, another
small, white-haired woman in a wheelchair. I look from Old
Frances to Addie and back again trying to find differences in
their faces so I can remember who is who. It's hard. Why is it
so hard? All of a sudden, I realize how unaccustomed I am to
actually looking at the elderly. All little old white-haired ladies
look the same to me. I have to concentrate. I begin to see: Old
Frances is smaller and bonier. Addie has big, surprised-looking
blue eyes.

After breakfast, it's time to toilet everyone. Part of the personal
care the facility promises to provide is toileting the residents
every two hours. This can be as blessedly simple as reminding
someone that it's time to go to the bathroom—so-called cueing
(only a few residents are able to function with this minimal
help)—or as labor-intensive as lifting a resident out of a wheelchair and holding her up while another RA (wearing gloves) rips
off her diaper and assesses and deals with whatever is there.
Then the two caregivers steer the resident to the toilet seat, sit
her down, turn on the faucet for inspiration, and pray for something. Whatever goes in the pot doesn't go in the diaper, which
means an easier change next time. Because each neighborhood
has only one caregiver on shift, Frances would normally have to
use her walkie-talkie to call for the "Float"—the one part-time
extra caregiver who helps wherever needed—to accomplish
these two-person assists. But Jasmine and I are here today.

We start with Old Frances, who would be a two-person
assist—that is, she is wheelchair-bound and needs total care—
except that she weighs only ninety pounds, so one caregiver can
handle her alone. When we wheel her into her room, I notice

something I had not noticed earlier: a handwritten sign taped to the wall that reads "Hospice patient. DO NOT CALL 9-1-1." I ask about this. Apparently, Old Frances has pretty much stopped eating, and her family and her doctor think the end is near. Her designation as hospice patient is a kind of death watch. No extraordinary measures will be taken to keep Frances alive. She'll get what's called palliative care, only what is needed to keep her comfortable. She is what is known in the world of eldercare as a "DNR"—do not resuscitate. I take a good long look at Old Frances. For an old, shriveled, demented, wheelchair-bound lady, she actually doesn't look too bad. It's hard to imagine that she's near death. But how would I know? Back in those much-vaunted days of extended families when women died in childbirth in their own beds, and children died of scarlet fever in their own beds, and grandma or grandpa, who lived with you, worked until they dropped right in front of you, people knew what death looked like. Not today. I have never seen a dead person, or a dying one.

Back out in the common area, Hayes is yelling for help again. Jasmine goes over to him. His arms are crossed over his chest. "Are you cold, Hayes?" she asks. It seems impossible given that he's wearing three layers of clothing, that it's a scorching August day, and that the neighborhood is kept at hot-house temperatures. "Are you hot?" she asks. He doesn't answer, doesn't seem to be paying any attention. "Are you just right?"

"Just right on the edge," says Hayes.

When lunch comes, I struggle again to get the right plates to the right people. I check and recheck the dietary list. I stare at Addie, then Old Frances, then back to Addie, still confused. Once I figure out who's who, I'm *still* confused. Is the lady I'm calling Old Frances Frances C. or Frances M.? I better not confuse them. Their dietary needs are quite different. I went through this just four hours ago at breakfast, but my mind's a blank. Why can't I keep this straight? Am *I* starting to have memory problems? This is, of course, not the first time I've had this thought. Every child of a parent with Alzheimer's secretly fears that there is a bad gene at work, a gene that's been passed on and lies in wait, ready to switch on the machinery of dementia when the time is right.

I know that early-onset Alzheimer's, a rare disease that hits a person in her fifties, or even forties, has a strong genetic link. But my mother's disease, coming in her seventies, was of the garden variety, the one that must be caused by *something* but no one knows what. If genes are implicated, the link is weak. Still, I wonder when my mother first suspected something was going wrong. Was she as young as I am now?

After lunch I am allowed a ten-minute break. Most of the other RAs spend their breaks and the thirty unpaid minutes we are allowed for lunch sitting outside, in an area behind the facility hidden by a tall fence, on sticky white plastic chairs where they chain-smoke and talk about their no-good boyfriends. I decide to take a pass. I grab my insulated Starbucks mug and get hot water from the kitchen to make a cup of tea. I brought the teabag from home, new fancy green tea I tried last month when my husband and I were at a spa resort. The box of fifteen teabags cost more than I make here in an hour. I sit on a Naugahyde banquette in the atrium massaging my legs and sipping tea.

I'm sure I can learn something from this place and these people, but I'm not sure what. I hope I have the strength and the stamina—physical and emotional—to stick around and find out. Right now it's all I can do to learn the job. I realize sitting here, six hours into my first day of on-the-job training, that I am no longer who I was just yesterday at orientation. I am not a reporter playing a role to get a story. I can't be. The work is too hard, too all-consuming. Helpless people depend on me. Here at Maplewood I am a caregiver, an RA like the other RAs, with a magnetic name tag clipped to my uniform shirt, with a walkie-talkie and a green half-apron stuffed with latex gloves. My job, for eight hours, is to care for people who can no longer care for themselves, who may no longer *be* themselves. My job is to be the good daughter.

At the end of the shift, sitting in my car in the parking lot, I take a moment to record in my reporter's notebook what we did, the three of us. This is what *one* of us will have to do—as in *me*—when the real work schedule begins next week:

11 people woken up, cleaned, and dressed
5 loads of laundry washed, dried, folded, and put in residents' rooms
11 people served breakfast
3 people hand-fed
kitchen cleaned
tables wiped and cleaned
2 people showered
8 people toileted three times
11 people served lunch
3 people hand-fed
kitchen cleaned
tables wiped and cleaned
carpet swept
garbage collected from 11 rooms and kitchen, taken out to Dumpster

I am glad it takes almost a half hour to drive home, an un-heard of commute in this town, because I need every minute of it. For the first fifteen minutes I obsess about the residents. I talk out loud, naming all the names I can remember, mentally going around the perimeter of the neighborhood, room by room, to see if I can match names with numbers: Marianne, 141; Eloise, 140; Hayes, 139. That's all I can do. I'll write myself a cheat sheet when I get home, a three-by-five file card I can stash in my half-apron next to the trash liners.

For the next fifteen minutes I try to ease myself through the transition from Maplewood into the world I know, the world I am comfortable with. It is a world of thoughts and ideas, of talk, of concepts, of books to be read and discussed, films to be seen. Diapers go on babies in my world.

The world I have just emerged from is entirely different: small, close, insular, tangible, unpredictable, earthy. This world is a series of disconnected intimate moments. Whatever happens happens when it wants to happen, not when you want it to. This world demands something different of you from moment to moment. I think of my life as the "real world" and Maplewood as something else. But maybe I'm wrong.

3

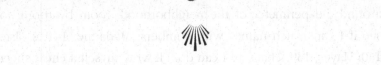

Anastasia, Frances's cousin, is our trainer today. She looks a lot like Frances, small, dusky-skinned, and moon-faced, but her attitude couldn't be more different. Frances talks about the residents, what they need, what we can do for them. Anastasia talks about the job, which she sees as an unending series of chores ranging from unpleasant to repugnant. Given what many of the chores are, she's got a point. But Frances somehow makes the work feel nurturing and intimate, like mothering or nursing. Anastasia makes it feel mindless and distasteful, like mucking out the stalls. "I don't want to be wiping asses my whole life," she tells Jasmine and me as we start the morning routine.

With every task Anastasia explains, each notation she makes in the comm log, every form she shows us, she adds, her voice a monotone: *If you don't do this, you'll get written up.* To get written up is the first step to losing the job. Her message to us is clear: You do the job not because you want to but because you have to. You do the job so you can keep the job—that is, until you find something better, something that pays more than minimum wage, something that doesn't involve wiping asses. When Jasmine and I are alone together in one of the resident's rooms making up a bed, we give each other pep talks to counter Anastasia's negativity. We're baffled over why she was given the responsibility of training us. Maybe because she's related to Calm Guam Frances the staff thinks she shares her cousin's Mother Teresa attitude toward the job. Or maybe, with C. G. Frances off today, and so few RAs who've been on the job for more than a few months, Anastasia was the only option. Whatever the reason, it was a mistake. If Jasmine and I didn't have each other today, one or both of us would be out the door.

At breakfast, I sit trying to feed Old Frances, tiny and birdlike with little faded blue eyes behind big glasses. I know from her file that she will be celebrating her ninety-eighth birthday this month. Ninety-eight is old, but somehow that number affects me less than realizing it means she was born in 1906. That was the year of the great San Francisco earthquake. Wyatt Earp was still alive. The Wright brothers were still tinkering. This feels like such ancient history—almost as inaccessible as the fall of the Roman Empire—that it's hard to connect it to the little woman in front of me. Frances's husband died in 1966. I am ashamed to say that my first thought is: Does that mean she hasn't had sex in thirty-eight years? I look at her and wonder. But sexual gratification, or lack thereof, is not Old Frances's top issue right now. Her immediate problem, the one I must address, is that she's stopped eating. She is the resident on hospice, the DNR. I have wheeled her out to the dining area anyway. Maybe today she'll eat. I kneel down by her chair and feed her a small bite of French toast. She chews and chews it, chews and chews it, doesn't swallow. Has she has forgotten that this is what you do when you have food in your mouth, that this is how you eat?

My mother was this way. I would arrive at her facility in time for lunch and spend the next two hours trying to feed her. Mostly she wouldn't open her mouth for me. Or if she did, she parted her lips but kept her jaw clamped shut. When I was able to sneak in a bite of something, she would chew and chew and chew. "Swallow," I would tell her. "Swallow," I would say, again and again, with increasing frustration, not willing to admit that she couldn't understand me. Maybe if I just said it one more time. Maybe if I said it louder. Maybe if I moved my face closer to hers. I would try to get her to drink something, thinking maybe the liquid in her mouth would force her to swallow.

I offer juice to Frances, and she rears back her head and clenches her teeth against the rim of the plastic cup. The movement is instantly familiar. My mother did this too. But with Frances, I find myself able to be philosophical: Maybe she knows she's at the end of her life and doesn't want to prolong the process of dying by taking in nourishment, I think. Maybe her body is busy shutting down and doesn't want to be interrupted. Maybe she is just elsewhere, otherwise engaged. There's a way of looking at Alzheimer's that is not about decline and loss but is instead about movement from the worldly to the spiritual. I heard someone talk about this at a conference. It's both wonderful and terrible to think these things as I try to feed Frances: wonderful because my reality shifts, and all of a sudden I feel myself in the presence not of a cantankerous old lady who's making my job harder by refusing to eat but instead embedded in an intimate moment that has more to do with end-of-life than with disease, more to do with transformation than with death, more to do with her than with me. But it's terrible, also, because it makes me realize how badly I handled the food thing with my mother. When she clenched her teeth against a spoon or fork or straw, I took it personally. She was rejecting my help.

She was rejecting my love. She was rejecting me. Why did I think that what she did was all about me?

Breakfast is over, but Hayes is not up yet. Anastasia has let him sleep until ten, which her cousin never would have done. Hayes is a lot of work, and Anastasia doesn't do anything she doesn't absolutely have to do. When we finally go into his room to wake him, we discover that he has wet his bed, soaked through his underwear and pajamas, his sheets and mattress pad. Jasmine and I get him out of bed and into the bathroom. He inches along behind his walker, asking us "what's next, what's next?" with every step. We strip off his soaked clothes and sit him on the toilet.

"You girls are so wonderful," he says. Hayes seems to know just when it's time to endear himself. "You are wonderful, too," says Jasmine. Hayes laughs his little dry laugh. "No, I'm not," he says. "I'm disgrummeled ... disgrinneled ... rummeled ..." "Grumpy?" Jasmine says, helping him along. He laughs.

But his mood changes immediately once he's seated at his usual spot at one of the smaller tables in the dining area. We re-heat his breakfast in the microwave and set it in front of him along with juice and milk. He is to have milk with every meal, his wife has ordered. When we turn away to do other tasks—it's time to toilet Addie and Old Frances; a woman named Pam who's connected to an oxygen tank needs help getting to her commode; there's laundry to be done—Hayes starts in with his "Help me, won't you please help me" litany. He needs some-one's full attention, and he knows how to get it. I sit with him and help him eat, talk to him, urge him on.

Anastasia says to finish up and get him back to his room. She says I should sit him in his big blue chair by the window and put on a CD. It must be eighty-five degrees in his room, and Hayes has on his usual set of long underwear under khakis, a long-sleeved shirt, and a sweater, but he asks for a blanket. He reminds me of General Sternwood, a character in Raymond Chandler's *The Big Sleep*. When private eye Philip Marlowe meets him, the old man is sitting bundled up in a wheelchair in the oppressive heat of an orchid greenhouse. "I seem to exist largely on heat, like a newborn spider," he tells Marlowe.

I put on a CD of the Tommy Dorsey band's greatest hits and hand Hayes a toy drum that sits on the floor next to the chair. He listens to the music and starts tapping out a beat, not the beat of the music, but a beat nonetheless. I thought that Anastasia was being cruel—or just lazy—about putting Hayes back in his room, that she was taking the easy way out. That may be true, but it is also a fact that Hayes is happier in his room, calmer. I watch as he stops tapping the drum, as his breathing gets deeper and slower, as his eyes close. It's been only a half hour since we woke him up, and he's asleep again. He'll doze in that chair until lunch.

Lunch for the RAs is sometime between 10:00 and 11:00 a.m., whenever the Float comes around to relieve us for our thirty minutes. We need to be back in plenty of time to get the residents ready for their noon meal. At 10:20, I clock out and look for a place to sit and eat the food I've brought from home in a plastic container. No one goes out to eat here. There's not enough time. There's no place within walking distance. At the tiny table in the windowless break room, the Hispanic woman who works as housekeeper is eating a giant-sized Cup O' Noodles and drinking a Big Gulp she brought with her, a meal I calculate at a thousand calories, plus or minus. A lot of the women who work here are big in that apple-shaped, broad-backed, ample-bosomed, pillowy way. After the first day of training when I got a sense of how physical the job was going to be, how many miles I would clock at work, I joked to Calm Guam Frances that I was sure I'd lose weight here. She smiled and told me she'd gained fifteen pounds.

A few steps from the break room is a door that leads to what might be called a patio—an eight-foot-square concrete slab furnished with a plastic picnic table, a soda machine, and a garbage can. You can smoke out here, so it is—despite the baking heat and the rank smell of refuse simmering in its own juices—a popular spot for lunch and breaks. Jasmine immediately lights up. I watch her smoke four cigarettes in less than fifteen minutes, lighting a new one from the butt of the old one, while Anastasia tells her about all the RAs who have quit or have been fired in the past month. I position myself upwind from the smoke, eat my lunch, and review the cheat sheet I keep tucked in my half-apron, the one with all the residents' names next to their room numbers. I'm halfway through day three, just four hours away from having to handle the neighborhood by myself, and I still don't have the names and room numbers memorized.

During the early afternoon, which is stressful but manageable with the three of us working together, Rose shuffles through the neighborhood. All the RAs know her. Rose is the most deeply demented resident at Maplewood. She has been here for as long as anyone can remember. But that doesn't mean much in a place with the impaired institutional memory that comes with high turnover. One administrator remembers back when Rose could talk, when she interacted with others, when she would look you in the eye. Now Rose lives in neighborhood 1, the unit with the lowest functioning folks, the ones in the advanced stages of the disease, but she is seldom in her own area. Unlike most of the residents, who stick close to home, she is restless, always moving. With the doors open between the neighborhoods all day, Rose goes where she pleases. Only sixty-eight years old, she is stoop-shouldered with short, unkempt, iron gray hair, a heavy, impassive face, and oddly frightening eyes that are simultaneously intense and lifeless. Unresponsive and unreachable, Rose spends her days wandering from one resident's room to another, pushing a chair or a walker in front of her, taking glasses or hearing aids, pillows, socks, knickknacks, whatever she can find, from one room and depositing them somewhere else.

It's a joke around here, I've already discovered. When anything is missing from anywhere—a clipboard from a locked cupboard, a coffee cup from the kitchen, Patty the receptionist's car keys, items that Rose could not possibly have access to—everyone says: "Rose took it." The RAs laugh, a kind of gallows humor, a way of humanizing Rose, incorporating her into the life of the facility. Otherwise, it's just too awful. Rose is very hard to handle and very hard to love, everyone's Alzheimer's nightmare. Casting her as a little gremlin helps diffuse the terror one feels being in her presence. Or maybe it's just the terror *I* feel.

I'm sure the RA in charge of her neighborhood dressed her in clean clothes this morning and combed her hair, but right now, Rose looks like she's been living in an alley for the past month. Her hair is wild, her clothes stained and rumpled. I see out of the corner of my eye that she is headed for Old Frances's room. I catch her just before she snatches a sweater from Frances's bed and walk her out to the common area. It's no good walking her back to her own neighborhood, Anastasia tells me. Don't bother, she says. Even if Rose will allow herself to be led, which is not likely, she'll be back in a few minutes.

A half hour later I discover Rose asleep on Hayes's bed. Hayes is sitting contentedly in his chair with his drum on his lap listening to Frank Sinatra sing "Fly Me to the Moon." Rose is

maybe three feet away, curled up with her hands pressed together prayerlike under her cheek. Hayes is oblivious. I call Jasmine in to take a look. We stand in the doorway chuckling.
Marianne, the resident who seems completely normal to me,
walks by and joins us. She thinks it's the funniest thing she's
ever seen. And then comes Anastasia. "We'll get written up if we
don't get Rose out of here," she says.

Later Anastasia tells me to go toilet Hayes by myself. When
she sees that I take the news in stride—after all, I'm a mother of
two sons—she adds that today is easy, but tomorrow and three
times each week, I will have to pull back Hayes's foreskin and
clean the head of his penis. That gets my attention. I maneuver
Hayes out of his big chair, inch him along to his bathroom, pull
down his khakis, long johns, and jockey shorts, inch him back
into position, and get him seated on the toilet. This takes close
to five minutes.

"Am I peeing?" he asks me. I listen carefully. It's hard to tell.
Peeing when you're ninety-one is not like peeing when you're
twenty-one or even fifty-one. It's a drippy faucet kind of pee.

"Yes," I say, "you are peeing."

"I keep peeing," he says. I pat him on the back for encour-
agement. "I'm dribbling. I'm dribbling," he says. It's true. "Am I
finished? Am I finished? My back itches."

Hayes goes from one thought to another without taking a
breath. Then, as if suddenly remembering his manners, as if suddenly remembering that someone is there caring for him, he turns
his handsome face up to me and says, "Thank you so much. You
are so kind."

On our "10"—one of the two ten-minute breaks we are supposed to (but sometimes don't) get during our shift—Jasmine
and I check the work schedule that's just been posted for the

month. She discovers that she is to start work the day after tomorrow, Sunday. We RAs have no control over which days we are scheduled to work, or which neighborhoods we are scheduled to work in. We can request a certain shift, but that too is at the behest of Christine, the Resident Care Coordinator, who has the impossible job of keeping all four neighborhoods staffed twenty-four hours a day, seven days a week, with a 60 to 70 percent staff turnover.

The problem with starting on Sunday is that Jasmine is a single mother, and she has no weekend childcare. She asks to use the phone in the reception area and calls whatever social service agency is helping her. Working full-time at minimum wage, Jasmine needs food stamps and a housing voucher to support herself and her son. She also gets a certain number of hours of childcare paid for, but she has to use the childcare providers on the agency's list.

She's put on hold, then transferred and put on hold again. Finally she gets to someone to explain the problem. I see Jasmine look at her watch. Seven of our ten allotted break minutes are gone. She asks Patty, the receptionist, if she can receive a fax—the list of approved childcare providers. After she gets off work today, she will start calling from the list. Maybe she can find someone who will take her son on a Sunday, beginning at 6:00 a.m., with a day's notice. If she does, she won't have the luxury of meeting this person beforehand, of checking out the house or the neighborhood. And that's the best-case scenario.

If she can't find childcare, she has to try to find someone to work her shift. But she's new here, like me, and has never done anyone a favor, never worked a shift for anyone else, so who, exactly, would be willing to do this for her? And what would it look like to Christine if a brand-new employee on her first day of real work finds a substitute instead of reporting for her shift?

If Jasmine asks for a change in the schedule, she has identified herself as a problem even before she starts working, and—as Anastasia would be first to point out—there's a good chance Jasmine would be fired.

So, on our one short break in the afternoon, the one time we can get out of the neighborhood, be by ourselves, close our eyes, put up our feet, or in Jasmine's case, grab a smoke or three, all she has done is traded the problems of the neighborhood for her own problems. I watch her, consumed with my own guilty secret: I am getting special treatment from Christine. I can schedule my own days. And not only can I work when I want, I can work where I want, in neighborhood 3.

The crisis of the afternoon is Jane's key. She can't find it anywhere. Jane is one of the most independent people in the neighborhood. Even tempered, invariably pleasant, and always calm, Jane is a little fire hydrant of a woman—a sturdy, squat 4 foot 11 with a round, open, expressive face that makes her look fifteen years younger than she proudly and correctly proclaims herself to be, which is eighty-eight. Jane dresses, bathes, and feeds herself. She likes to help clear dishes from the table. She has a stash of Tootsie Rolls in her room and often doles them out after mealtime. She sits and talks with many of the other women, listening when they spout nonsense, patting their hands, nodding sympathetically. She is clearly the social center of the neighborhood.

Jane has a sense of herself that most of the other residents in the neighborhood, farther advanced in their disease, do not. It is important, for example, for her to maintain her privacy, to have an uninvadable space that is her own. I think the key symbolizes whatever little independence she has left. Like Marianne, the other almost fully self-sufficient person in the neighborhood, she locks her door when she is not in her room. She always keeps her key on a squiggly plastic cord around her wrist. But it's not there.

She ransacks her room and can't find it. When she learns that the toilet is clogged in the bathroom she shares with the woman who lives next door, she decides that her neighbor must have taken her key and tried to flush it. That might sound a little paranoid, but weirder things have happened here, I am told. Jim the janitor comes in to unclog the toilet. No key.

Jane was so upset that she ate no lunch today, and Jane is a hearty eater. After I return from my 10, I tell Jane that I will help her look for the key, that we are sure to find it, that it cannot have gone far.

"Must be Rose," Jasmine says with a grin. I check every surface in the common area and scour her room. Nothing. She trails after me, looking more worried by the moment. I can't find the key, and I have no luck redirecting her attention. Some of the others who are more far gone are easy to redirect because their attention span is so short. Most of the other residents here would have already forgotten that something was missing.

An hour later, as I'm doing the last chores on my shift, I open the washing machine door to transfer Jane's clothes to the dryer. The squiggly plastic cord with her key falls out. I grab it and run to find her, brandishing the key above my head. When she sees me, her face lights up. It doesn't just light up, it transforms. She is elated and relieved and thankful and joyously happy, as if she had just been shown a newborn grandchild. She hugs me, the top of her head fitting nicely under my chin. She thanks me, again and again. It feels like I just saved her pet dog from a house fire or found a cure for cancer. Or Alzheimer's.

When I leave at 2:45, it is ninety-eight degrees outside. Across the street from Maplewood, one of the other day shift RAs is sitting on a concrete bench in the baking sun waiting for a bus to take her home. More than a few women who work here work here for a reason I never would have thought of: Maplewood is on a bus line. For them, a car, an operational vehicle, is a luxury, and the decision about where to be employed is dictated not by hourly wage or working conditions but by bus routes. I get in my car and crank up the air conditioner. I turn on the radio, loud. I want to drown out the voices that are telling me *you can't possibly do this.*

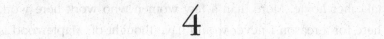

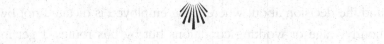

On the way to my first day of real work, my first day alone and in charge of neighborhood 3, I spend the first half of the pre-dawn commute talking myself down from panic. I tell myself what Calm Guam Frances told me: *Just get in there and establish a routine, find your own rhythm.* But there is so much to do, so many chores, so many details, so many people depending on me, that the advice feels like an aphorism, not a plan. What I need is a plan. So I walk myself through the day, chore by chore, resident by resident.

I'll read the comm log first, of course, to see how everyone has been doing since I was last in the neighborhood three days ago. I'll check the S/L schedule to see who needs showers. Then I'll start the wake-up routine. Who first? Someone easy like Jane to build my confidence, or someone difficult like the delusional, contentious Frances M. to get the worst over with quickly? I think I need to just jump in. I'll start with Frances M. Then I'll go to Old Frances, who is generally compliant but needs total care. That will take a while. Next I'll give myself a break and wake up

Eloise, who is already one of my favorites. She'll be easy. Then I'll call for help with Addie, the two-person assist. Better get to Hayes next. I can do this, I tell myself.

It matters that I do this job well. The residents depend on me. Their world is very small now, the rooms and corridors of Maplewood, and I am in charge of it all. What is left to them is the warm, dry clothes I dress them in, the cup of coffee I offer, the tape of *I Love Lucy* I put in the VCR, the hug as I pass by to do another chore. What is left, because it is so little, takes on great significance. And so I want, and need, to do these many small things well. The families depend on me, just as I and my family depended on the women who cared for my mother.

And the families pay a lot for this care. I may be making minimum wage, but the cost of putting a family member into one of the twenty-five hundred or so specialized memory care facilities nationwide, many of which, like Maplewood, are part of vast eldercare chains, is considerable. The yearly price tag (exclusive of medical expenses, of course) can range from $30,000 to more than $100,000, depending on geography, amenities, and, most important, level of care.

At Maplewood, as elsewhere, each resident has what's called a "service plan," a multipage document that details what help the person needs to accomplish the simple daily activities of life. Can the person get out of bed in the morning? Dress herself? Brush her own teeth? Is the person able to walk? Is she incontinent? Can she feed herself? Maplewood's service plan is an itemized list that covers thirty-one categories, from "mobility," "dressing," and "personal hygiene" to "transportation" and "medication." The language is straightforward and clinical, but the subtext is fraught with emotion. Here, in black and white, is the diminution of life, the slow ebb of self-reliance, the progressive loss of independence. Here, also, in exact detail, is the cost of care—because the more care needed, the more it will cost the family. At Maplewood the amount of the monthly bill is based on a point system. Each activity—showering, toileting, dressing, eating—is quantified according to how much help the resident needs, from 0 points—no help at all—to 20 points, which is considered "extended care."

The details are all worked out at a conference between the family and Maplewood staff when the resident first comes here. At the meeting, which is at once intimate and impersonal, all categories are discussed and evaluated, after which the "service points" (the 0 to 20 range for each activity) are totaled to determine the level of care: level 1 is 0 to 50 points total; level 4, the highest, is anything higher than 151 points. Each level carries a progressively higher price tag. Jane, fully mobile and independent, is charged the lowest rate—at Maplewood, about $40,000 a year. Old Frances and Addie, in wheelchairs, need help with everything. The cost to their families is $52,000.

The system, with its itemized categories, its precise allocation of points, and its crisp statistical certainty, fools you into thinking it works. But I wonder. After my third day of training last week, I spent an extra hour (unpaid) reading through the black binder that is the collection of my residents' service plans.

I turned first to Frances M.'s because I think of her as the most difficult to care for person in the neighborhood, the most unpredictable. She is the one who wakes up in the middle of the night and pees on the carpet. She is the one who undresses herself after you dress her, and then undresses herself again after you dress her again. She would need the highest level of care, I figured.

At the beginning of the plan is a summary of Frances M.'s medical conditions. She has an underactive thyroid, very low blood pressure, osteoporosis, and Parkinson's. And, of course,

Alzheimer's. The body is such a complicated machine, so many parts, so many systems, so many opportunities for errors and breakdowns. It's a wonder it all works, so I guess it's not surprising when ultimately, it doesn't. As I read Frances's chart, I thought about Nanny, my mother's mother. At Frances M.'s age, mid-eighties, Nanny got on a plane and flew a thousand miles to be at my wedding. Into her nineties she was mobile, continent, coherent, and feisty. She could see. She could hear. She was interested in life. Then one day, at ninety-four, her worst ailments being dry eyes and diverticulitis, she died at home in bed. I must keep reminding myself as I look at Frances M.'s plan, as I work here changing diapers and spoon-feeding, that there are other ways life can end. There's Nanny's way.

As I studied Frances M.'s service plan a few days ago, I was struck by the difference between the person I was reading about and the person I had been caring for in the neighborhood. The person in the service plan needed only "cueing" (which adds zero points) to get up and out in the morning. But the real Frances M. needs to be coaxed out of bed not just once but many times. She needs to be dressed, not *cued* to get dressed. When I put toothpaste on her brush and handed it to her the other morning, she stood there, frozen, holding the toothbrush in her hands, eyes at half-mast, muttering. She often freezes in place. It must be the Parkinson's. I started brushing her teeth. Then she took over and wouldn't stop. I couldn't get her to stop. She was making her gums bleed, and she wouldn't stop. I had to wrench the toothbrush out of her hand. So much for cueing to brush teeth.

Maybe the difference between Frances M. on paper and Frances M. in the flesh is wishful thinking on her daughter's part, or perhaps denial. It's easy to imagine that Deanne, Frances M.'s cheerful, sweet-faced daughter, can't admit to herself just how far gone her mother is. She may not even see it. It's also easy to understand why a relative might *purposely* underestimate the care needed, not that I think this is what Deanne did. But, in fact, the less care listed in the service plan, the less the monthly expense. Of course, in the trenches, where I am, it makes no difference how much someone's family is paying. If Deanne isn't paying for the correct level of care for Frances M., her mother gets the care she needs anyway.

Whatever happens, Maplewood wins. If a relative does pay the higher rate for extended care, the facility makes more money, none of which goes to increasing the wages of the people who do the extra work. But if a relative doesn't pay for the care, Maplewood's bottom line doesn't suffer. We RAs do the work anyway, for the same hourly wage.

But I can't, and don't, think of it this way. My minimum-wage work at Maplewood may pay less than any job I've had since I reshelved books in the library as a college freshman, but it demands more personal responsibility than any other job I've ever had, unless motherhood counts. I want to do it well. In fact, I want to excel. Maybe it's because I want to excel in everything I do, or maybe it's because I am trying to compensate for not excelling with my mother. I don't know. But really, how hard can it be, I think to myself as I drive in to work. All these other women do this job. If they can do it, surely I can do it. This is what I tell myself at 6:20 a.m. as I pull into the parking lot in front of Maplewood.

I clock in a few minutes early, stash my lunch in the mini-fridge, load up my apron with latex gloves, clip on the walkie-talkie, and read through the comm log. Then I take a deep breath and make my way to Frances M.'s room. I have seen how obstinate and combative and utterly unreachable she can be. The first morning I trained in the neighborhood, she yelled at me and refused to get up. The second morning, after Jasmine and I spent fifteen minutes tending to her and getting her dressed, she scurried back to her room, undressed herself, and went back to bed the moment we moved on to the next resident.

Frances M. talks a lot. She mutters and mumbles and babbles. During the three days of training, I at first couldn't make much sense of it, but then I began to focus in and I picked up on recurring words and themes. She was apparently talking about school, about elementary school. She seemed to be back at the time when one of her now fifty-something daughters was a third grader. "Is school over?" she asked me once. "Are you the teacher's aide?" At the time I was trying, unsuccessfully, to get her to eat. Then I had a brainstorm. Maybe I could break through and communicate with her if we were in the same moment, her moment. I told her that she better eat her lunch because school would be out pretty soon, and she would need to go pick up her daughter. Frances nodded and proceeded to eat her entire lunch. Jasmine looked over in wonder. After lunch, I told Frances that I was the teacher and that she could be my assistant that afternoon. For the next hour, she followed me around calmly, helping as I loaded laundry, delivered clean clothes to residents' rooms, put in a new video. Then I read from the posted menu.

"This is what the cafeteria will be serving," I told her. I was being so clever. She took a good look around the common area where the other residents were sitting.

"These students are pretty old," she said.

But whatever key I thought I had discovered to moderating Frances M.'s behavior is not unlocking anything today. I try every possible iteration of the school idea, but Frances will have none of it. She kicks at me when I try to pull down her covers. She tells me to go to hell when I tell her it's time for school, that her daughter is dressed and ready, that the bus will be leaving soon. I've been at it for more than ten minutes and have accomplished nothing. The more frustrated I become, the more agitated she becomes.

At the Alzheimer's conference I went to, the experts talked about this. They think that those with this disease might develop a hypersensitivity to the emotional states of those around them, a kind of elevated emotional intuition to compensate for their diminished cognitive skills. That means that at least sometimes those scary unwanted behaviors—agitation, violence, verbal abuse—are actually a reflection of the fear and agitation of the caregiver. At home, when it's your husband or wife, your father or mother, and you are scared and sad and frustrated and coping all alone, it's easy to see how the behaviors can escalate. Here I take a deep breath, walk out of Frances M.'s room, and go on to the next person on my wake-up list.

But first I check on Ella. She is a large, silent woman with a curiously unlined face who mostly keeps to herself. I haven't had much chance to interact with her yet. I don't know much about her other than she likes to sleep late. In her service plan, it says not to wake her until eleven. But she's been known to get up before then, and she's not steady on her feet (also in her service plan), so I am to check on her every ten minutes all morning. She's asleep and snoring when I peek in her room. I go on to Addie, who needs a shower this morning. With the help of the roving extra RA known as the Float, I get Addie out of bed, undressed, showered, shampooed, dressed, and in her wheelchair in record time. Ella is still asleep when I check. I wake up Eloise and help her dress. Back to Ella, who is still asleep. Then it's Marianne and Jane, who just need to be told that breakfast will be served soon. They can take care of themselves. I stop to pour Eloise a cup of decaf. I go to check on Ella again. This time she isn't in her bed. Her room smells awful.

In the bathroom I find Ella sitting on the floor, her back against the tiled wall, her legs splayed in front of her, her nightgown hiked to her waist. Her face is beaded with sweat, and she is bleeding from a small cut on the side of her head. I look at her, and my mouth goes dry. I look at her, and in slow motion, at a pace I want to but can't control, I take in the whole scene. She is sitting in a pool of diarrhea. Her legs are slathered with it. There are wet brown skid marks on the floor. I feel clammy in the small of my back. Nothing makes sense until everything does: Ella awoke sometime between my ten-minute checks, walked to the bathroom, didn't make it all the way to the toilet, and slipped and fell in her own shit.

I can't move. I can't think. A rivulet of sweat is running down the back of my leg. It's just me and Ella, and we're both senseless. But then something happens, some delayed adrenaline rush, and I am suddenly in overdrive, suddenly more focused, more in the moment than I can ever remember being. I grab the walkie in my apron pocket.

"This is neighborhood 3," I say. I keep my voice calm. "I need help immediately with . . ." I can't remember Ella's room number. I'm not supposed to use her name on the walkie-talkie. In my apron pocket is the cheat sheet. I fish around for it, grab it . . . "with 132. I'm in the bathroom. Immediately."

I kneel down beside Ella and talk to her. I tell her everything is okay. I hold her hand. This close to the floor, I am woozy from the smell. Before I can do anything else, Calm Guam Frances and Tiffany, the Med Aide on duty, both arrive. Quickly, Tiffany takes Ella's vitals, which are normal. She asks Ella to wiggle her toes, bend her knees, move her legs, but Ella doesn't understand, so very carefully, Tiffany does it for her. Everything seems to be okay. The cut on her forehead is superficial. She'll have a headache and a goose egg. That could be the extent of it, but

Tiffany can't be sure. She calls the main desk on her walkie and asks Patty to call for the EMTs. Ella needs to go to the hospital to be checked out.

As we wait for the ambulance, we begin the task of cleaning her up, grabbing washcloths and wipes, swabbing down her legs, covering the mess on the floor with towels so none of us will slip and fall. We work within inches of each other, within inches of Ella. We are silent and sweating. We need to get her into the shower, but when the three of us work together to haul her to her feet and get her positioned with her walker, we see immediately that she cannot support her own weight. She is in pain. Tiffany grabs a wheelchair, and we gently lower her to the seat. Her groin and buttocks and back are still coated with shit. We wheel her into the shower: warm water, soap, three washcloths, six hands. We wheel her out, pat her dry, dress her carefully in a clean nightgown. When we're finally finished and standing around the wheelchair, sweating and silent, Calm Guam Frances rests her small brown hand on my shoulder. I want to lean into her. I want her to tell me it's not my fault. I want to cry. A few minutes later, the EMTs come, load Ella on a gurney, and take her away.

What I'd like to do now is take a long walk or sit quietly with a cup of tea, think things through, decompress. But that's not how this job works. I have been with Ella forty-five minutes, which means that breakfast is now late. It was delivered a half hour ago and is sitting on the cart getting cold. I walk out into the common area and get back to work. I check the dietary schedule for who is allergic to eggs, who gets finger food, whose food has to be diced in small pieces, and I start serving. I leave the cream of wheat cereal on the lower shelf for the moment. It's already cold and rubbery. When I jiggle the bowl, the cereal slides side to side in one bowl-shaped piece. I have never seen any resident actually eat the hot cereal that is part of breakfast every day. As I'm pouring coffee, Cathy, the Float, a rode-hard-and-put-away-wet woman who is probably fifteen years younger than me but looks twenty years older, takes a look at the un-served cereal bowls and starts yelling at me. I tell her that residents don't seem to like hot cereal and that it's ice-cold anyway. She tells me she's been working here a lot longer, and she knows better—a point well taken, just not at this moment and not at this decibel.

"I'm going to tell Christine," she says, storming off. I am being reported. Just as Cathy leaves, Susan, the activities director, rushes in. She looks around, doesn't say hello.

"There's no music," she says, accusingly. "You need to have a video or music on at all times."

I go on my ten-minute break and try to find someplace to be alone. The break room is tiny and airless. The little table is covered in crumbs. I can smell the meat cooking in the industrial kitchen across the hall. I open the door to the back area with the plastic picnic table, hoping no one is out there. But Lena is, another of the RAs. She is a tough, sharp-tongued woman who is universally disliked. I move to go back inside, but she tells me to come join her. I can't think of how to say no. I can't think at all. I sit on a hot plastic chair and watch Lena light a new cigarette from the butt of her old cigarette, and I start to sob. Lena smokes and watches.

I tell her about Ella because I need to tell someone. She tells me story after story about people who have fallen and died, people who have choked and died, a woman she found in bed who had bled to death. I think this is supposed to make me feel better. I stop listening and start glancing at my watch. This ten-minute break has already lasted twelve minutes. I try to break away twice before I manage to leave her there, in the hot sun, lighting another cigarette. Her mother, she tells me as I walk away, died of emphysema and lung cancer.

When I get back to neighborhood 3, Cathy is there with a hard glint in her eye. "Ten minute breaks are supposed to be ten minutes," she says. "I'm telling Christine."

Some people think of those who suffer from Alzheimer's as little children, as babies, because they have to be dressed and fed and toileted. But they're not. Babies love your touch. Babies learn. For Hayes, every time I take him to the bathroom is the first time. He doesn't remember from ten o'clock to noon to two o'clock, even though the process is exactly the same. "What next?" he says, when I steer his walker through the bathroom door. "What next?" he asks, between each mini-step. "Can I sit yet? Can I sit yet?" he asks, when we are halfway to the toilet. When he is finally seated, I need to tell him, three or four times, that he is on the toilet and that it is okay to pee.

This afternoon, all that accomplished once again, Hayes, sitting with his three layers of clothes puddled at his feet, lets out a grunt. I hear something plop into the toilet. "My, that was a BIG one," he says, proudly. He is so pleased with himself that I cannot help but be pleased too. The simple pleasure of evacuation. We grin at each other. Then I maneuver him back to his big chair, put on some music, hand him his toy drum, and tell him I'll be back to get him in a few minutes for lunch. As soon as I walk out, he starts yelling.

"What do you need?" I ask him, turning back. He looks at me quizzically. I think he's forgotten he just yelled.

"Why don't you take a little nap before lunch?" I suggest.

"Can I go to sleep?" he asks. "Can I go to sleep?"

"Yes."

"I won't get lost?"

"No," I say. "You won't get lost. Anyway, Hayes, I'll find you."

Later, at lunch, he is carrying on as usual, waving his fork and yelling for help, yelling for someone to "Come here, come closer, come here now." But I am right next to him, busy loading his spoon with diced mystery meat and overcooked squash. Where is he that he doesn't realize I'm at his elbow? Doesn't he see me?

"Hayes," I say, speaking more to myself than him, "Hayes, if I were any closer I'd be on top of you."

"Ha-ha-ha," he says, laughing his precise, staccato, dry laugh. It actually *sounds* like ha, ha, ha. "You are so funny. You are such a funny lady." Wherever he was, he came back in time to get the joke.

As I am leaving for the day, Brooke tells me she's heard from the hospital. The fall in the bathroom broke Ella's hip. That's what the X-rays showed. There will be no surgery. Ella's children have ordered palliative care only.

I drive to the athletic club, work out hard for an hour and a half, take a long shower, lather three times with aromatherapy Aveda body wash, shampoo my hair even though it's clean, and dress in a new T-shirt I buy at the front desk because I can't stand the thought of putting on my Maplewood uniform shirt. I can still smell Ella. After dinner, my husband and I go for a walk, and I tell him about Ella. He tells me that some things are beyond my control. This is not what a woman with Sun, Mercury, Venus, and Mars in Aries likes to hear. Or can understand.

"But that's my job," I tell him. "My job is to make sure nothing bad happens to anybody."

5

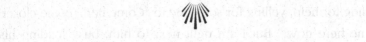

Susan is Maplewood's "life engagement coordinator," a fanciful title that at first turns me off. It is, I think, inflated, akin to calling a sales clerk a "customer service associate." Susan is the activities director. Why not just keep the nomenclature simple? But the more time I spend here, the more I see what she does, the more I appreciate the grander title.

Susan is a built-for-comfort, henna-haired, extravagantly perky woman in her mid-fifties. She has formed such an emotional attachment to the residents here that when she married the retired minister who comes in to lead weekly "spirit sings," she staged a complete re-creation of their wedding ceremony in the common area of neighborhood 3 so the residents could all be part of it. She had it videotaped too. I saw the tape—Susan pressed it on me the first time we met, back when I was observing here, not working—and it is so heartwarming that you get overheated. Susan cries every time she watches the tape, which is often enough to be a little weird.

It's Susan's job to keep things interesting at Maplewood, to make each day a little different. One afternoon she might organize a birthday party, the next, bring in a baby lamb for a visit. She's big on animals: bunnies, chicks, cats, dogs, birds, even a full-grown, toilet-trained llama named Camas. She plans concerts and sing-alongs, van rides, and ice-cream socials, special movie nights with popcorn, occasional afternoons spent listening to old radio shows on tape, exercise classes, and, several times a week, a game called balloon ball. She's here in neighborhood 3 this morning, walkie-talkying to the RAs in the other neighborhoods, entreating them to send over their residents for the activity. It takes a while—everything takes a while here—but Susan is a persistent woman. I help by corralling a half-dozen of my residents, sweet-talking Eloise and agreeable Jane and a few others, wheeling in Old Frances, then returning to my chores, one of which, my favorite, is putting a batch of sugar cookies in the oven. This is Susan's idea too. She wants the neighborhoods to smell sweet and doughy.

In the activity area next to the kitchen, Susan has set out fifteen chairs in a wide circle. Residents from all four neighborhoods, coaxed, cajoled, and accompanied by their RAs, are settling in. Today's Float, an unfamiliar face, stands in the middle of the circle and taps a big red vinyl balloon ball high in the air, directing it toward Jack, a guy from neighborhood 4. The idea of the game is to keep the ball in play, in the air, with the staffer batting it first to one resident, then another, each one returning the ball with a healthy whack. The activity combines physical exercise, hand-eye coordination, concentration, and a bit of socializing. From a life engagement perspective, it is a winner. But, from my vantage point in the kitchenette, I can't imagine how this is going to work, how, between the infirmities and slow reflexes of old age, and the disconnect of Alzheimer's, these men and women are going to keep the ball in the air. Or have fun.

Jack, from neighborhood 4, is a compact, alert-looking fellow. He is sitting protectively close to a wispy-haired redhead named Caroline. They don't look at each other, but their knees are touching. Jack doesn't seem to be watching the ball, but when it drifts over to him, he taps it gingerly in the direction of this guy named Dan. But Dan is not paying attention at all. Maybe he's daydreaming of the fishing trips he used to take. He was quite a fisherman. Or the long, sunny days he spent at the coast after he retired. Or maybe his switch is just flipped in the off position. Earlier that morning, when I was in his neighborhood to borrow kitchen supplies from the RA there, he invited me into his room to show me his oil paintings, simple landscapes he rendered in his retirement years. The walls of his room are his gallery. I admired the paintings, nodding my head as he struggled to explain them to me.

"You see the"—he paused, working hard—"the . . . the . . . thing?" There was a wooden shed in the foreground of the painting we were looking at, which was what I thought he might mean.

"Yes, I see it," I told him, and he seemed to be relieved not to have to explain anymore. Then he touched my elbow lightly and guided me to the next painting, a dramatic seascape. We looked at it silently, and I smiled at him, and I thought, We are having a Moment, this man and I. This is just what I hoped for when I took the job. Then Dan turned his back to me, pulled down his pants and boxers so they bunched around his ankles, and shuffled over to the bathroom, leaving me to contemplate his skinny white rear end. I deemed the Moment officially over and left him to his business.

Now Dan is sitting straight in his seat with a dreamy look in his eyes. But when the balloon ball connects with his bald head, he is suddenly alive. He lets out a big laugh. The joke is on him, and he gets it. Jane laughs. The woman across the circle whose name I don't know yet laughs. Dan grabs the ball and bats it over to a wizened old lady, who is slumped over in her wheelchair snoring softly.

"Tilda, wake up. We're playing." The Float puts the ball in Tilda's lap, but Tilda isn't interested. The ball drifts to the floor. The Float tries to rouse Tilda one more time before picking up the ball and starting the play anew. She taps the ball to the opposite side of the circle where a lively, good-natured woman named Dottie is sitting, her chair pulled close to Eloise's. Dottie, who lives in the room next to Eloise and considers her a special friend, used to play volleyball in high school, and whatever else she may have forgotten—her children's names, where she used to live, her age—she has not forgotten how to serve a ball. She curls in the fingers of her right hand, cocks her arm and raises it high, then brings the heel of her hand down hard on the ball. It whizzes across the full diameter of the circle. A sweet old man in baggy jeans, a visitor from neighborhood 4, sees it just in time and gets a piece of it.

"San Francisco!" Dan yells, apropos of nothing. The ball heads over to Tilda again, but this time she's awake and ready. She plays it cagey, though, letting the ball settle by her feet and then giving it a kick, a bit too vigorously, in the direction of the sweet old man in baggy jeans. He's right there, batting it back to Tilda, hard. Susan, on the periphery of the circle, sees something is brewing.

"Tilda," she says, walking over and putting a hand on the old lady's shoulder, "let's go get a glass of water." By the time Tilda returns to the circle two minutes later, both she and the old man in the baggy jeans have forgotten their incipient tiff. The game, meanwhile, is in full swing. Jack, Dan, Dottie, and a pretty little woman with big glasses and a thatch of white hair are the major players, but everyone, from time to time, joins in. They are more agile than I thought they would be, bending over to retrieve a ball that's settled between their legs, getting up from the chair to grab a ball that's sailed over their heads, kicking, swatting, batting. And laughing. They laugh at their own efforts, successful and un-. They laugh when Dan spaces out again, and the ball connects with his shiny forehead. They laugh when Jack tries to get Caroline to hit the ball and instead she gives him a you-have-a-nice-time-dear-but-leave-me-out-of-it look. They laugh when Dottie serves so hard that the ball drifts halfway to the kitchen.

I am watching the action as carefully as I can while also tending to the sugar cookies in the oven, keeping juice glasses and coffee cups refilled for the residents lingering at the dining room table, and finding the odd moment to scribble in the reporter's notebook I keep next to my supply of latex gloves in the pocket of my half-apron. I want to get down all the details so I can later reconstruct the scene and make this observed moment come alive.

I move to the other side of the kitchen counter, closer to the circle of chairs, notebook in hand. Just then, the ball comes sailing my way. Dottie has given it a mighty *thwap* from the other side of the circle. I have just enough time to drop the notebook and give the ball a whack before it drifts to the floor. I direct it to Jack, who taps it back to me. I tap it to Caroline, but she lets Jack get it, so I tap it to her again. She gives me a look. Jack pats her cheek, grabs the ball, and keeps it in play. Meanwhile, the Float, who had been coordinating the game from the center of the circle, catches a glimpse of a resident struggling with her walker and rushes to help her. Without thinking, I move in to take her place before the ball can touch the ground. Alone at the center, I *whap* the ball to Dottie, who laughs at my imitation of her. Dan takes a turn. Tilda is back in the game. Even Old Frances, old Do-Not-Resuscitate Frances, is smiling, alert, following the game with her eyes. Something is going on here, something vibrant and alive.

I'm into it now. I see if we can keep the ball in the air for ten successive taps. (Yes!) I see if I can get everyone to hit the ball at least once. (Almost.) I see if we can keep *two* balls, the red one and a yellow one sitting forgotten next to Old Frances's wheelchair, in the air simultaneously. (We can't.) I have forgotten the reporter's notebook. I have forgotten the need to record this. I am working up a sweat, and, like the fifteen people around me in the circle this morning, I am living the moment. *This is fun.*

6

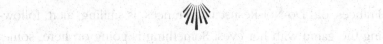

A few days later, Susan bustles in with the news that she has set up a nursery in neighborhood 1. She is very proud and wants me to take a look. On my ten-minute break I go across the atrium to the other neighborhood, an exact replica of my neighborhood, but populated with residents more deeply demented, more out of touch with reality, than the folks in my charge. Susan has commandeered a nook in the large common area, furnishing it with a crib, chest of drawers, and rocking chair. Above the crib is a bunny mobile. On top of the chest of drawers are four stuffed teddy bears and a stack of picture books. Everything is done up exactly as it would be in a baby's room: the crib has a duck-themed quilt, bumper, and dust ruffle; there are diapers and baby clothes in all the drawers; a stack of receiving blankets is draped across the arm of the rocking chair.

But there are no babies here. Or rather, there are no real babies. That's not quite right either: there are five baby-dolls that five residents in neighborhood 1 *think* are real. They care for them as if they are real, dressing them, swaddling them, holding them, rocking them, cooing at them, putting them down for naps. These women who no longer have the ability to regulate their own lives—they cannot dress themselves; they do not know when mealtime is or when to go to bed—somehow effortlessly keep their baby-dolls on a predictable daily schedule. These women who have forgotten the names of their real children and who could not find their way from the dining room table back to their own rooms at Maplewood, remember where they put their dolls for naptime and every day, after lunch, remember to retrieve them.

This baby-doll phenomenon is not unique to Maplewood. I saw the same thing—minus the beautifully furnished nursery—at my mother's Alzheimer's facility. It took some getting used to. In fact, I thought it was downright creepy when I first saw these old women hugging and rocking plastic dolls. I felt as if I'd walked into an episode of *The Twilight Zone*. My reaction, Susan tells me, is a common one. Relatives who visit and see Mom or Grandma gazing lovingly into the polymer eyes of a Toys "Я" Us special are disconcerted, saddened, and just plain weirded out. The whole baby-doll thing is frowned upon by some in the Alzheimer's care community, as well as those in state agencies set up to oversee eldercare facilities, because they worry—and rightly so—about "infantilizing" the elderly. People who suffer from Alzheimer's may seem to regress to childhood or even infancy. Their language skills erode and then disappear. They lose the ability to care for themselves. They end their days wearing diapers. But they are not children, and they should not be treated as such, caution those in the care community. Allowing them to play with dolls is treating them like children. What this logical and laudably respectful position fails to take into consideration is that these women are not playing with dolls. In the Alzheimer's-induced altered state in which they live, they are caring for real infants.

It all started in neighborhood 1 when a new resident began carting a doll with her to mealtimes. It was a very old doll from her childhood, the kind with glass eyes and a painted ceramic face. Her relatives had brought it in, along with much decorative memorabilia, to make her room homier, more familiar. When she put the doll down on a chair one day, another resident took it and squirreled it away in her room. A tiff ensued, and the RA back then, a big, kindhearted linebacker of a woman named Cindy, suggested to the second resident's family that they buy her her own doll. Now there were two women carting around dolls. Cindy noticed that the two of them began sitting next to each other on the couch, that they smiled at each other, that they began to ask about each other's "babies."

She also noticed that the most difficult woman in the neighborhood, a short-tempered combative lady named Billie, took a particular interest in the women with the dolls. Billie could not stand to be touched, which made caring for her difficult and frustrating. "Leave me alone," she'd yell at Cindy when the RA tried to guide her to the table for dinner. "Get away from me," she'd yell when Cindy tried to brush her teeth. Maybe, Cindy thought, if Billie touched something, held something, had something to care for, it might make a difference. She told the family who, somewhat incredulously, went out and bought her a doll.

I had met and gotten to know Cindy before I started work here, when I was still observing. She was a deeply empathetic but refreshingly plainspoken woman who had worked in nursing homes since she was eighteen—she was now in her early forties—with only a two-year break in all that time during which she made her living as a long-haul trucker. Funny, insightful, and no-nonsense, she thought she knew more about Alzheimer's care than the people who ran Maplewood. Observing in her neighborhood day after day, I couldn't help but agree.

With a baby-doll in her arms, Billie became a different person. She began to socialize, choosing to sit at the same table as the other two doll mothers. She lost her sharp tongue and instead spent afternoons humming and singing to the doll. She bounced the doll on her knee and rubbed its back. She smiled. When Billie resisted Cindy's ministrations, as she often still did, Cindy would kneel down next to her and smile at the doll. "What a lovely baby," Cindy would say, and like magic, Billie would calm down. One day I watched the three doll mothers sitting around a table, three women who had been lost in their private worlds. They were trading baby clothes, dressing and undressing their dolls, wrapping them, burping them, occasionally commenting to each other. They looked happy.

There's so much research about the medical aspects of Alzheimer's, the decoding of the disease, the amyloid plaques and neurofibrillary tangles, the push to diagnose early, the race to develop drugs to cure it or at least mitigate the symptoms. But there is little research, almost no attention given, to the *experience* of the disease, what day-to-day life is like for someone with Alzheimer's. The world they inhabit is like a foreign culture, one that can make little sense from the outside. RAs like Cindy are the unschooled, underpaid cultural anthropologists who immerse themselves in this new culture, and if they care and are bright like Cindy, they begin to make sense of it. Cindy no longer works at Maplewood—she lasted seven months, a considerable tenure in this trade—but she started something important. Susan, creator of the neighborhood 1 nursery, continues the work.

This morning in the nursery, one lady is sitting in the rocking chair, rocking her doll back and forth, back and forth, her eyes half-closed, her lips upturned in a half-smile. She has that dreamy look mothers have when they rock their babies. At one of the dining room tables sit Billie and two other doll mothers, all holding their swaddled babies to their chests. I watch as another resident, a spry little lady with an impish face, walks up to the table.

"How are the babies doing this morning?" she asks the women. They are not talkers. Words come to them slowly and with increasing difficulty. But they look up from their babies and smile. "Oooh, she is so cute," says the spry lady, reaching out to touch the head of Billie's doll. "And this one," she says, moving on to a baby swaddled in blue, "what a little tiger." As she walks away, she gives me a big wink. She knows, but she plays along anyway.

When I arranged for my mother to come West for part of what would be the last year of her life, my daughter, the third of my three children, was just four months old. Lizzie was an extraordinarily pretty baby, blue-eyed and rosy-cheeked with wisps of honey blond hair and that peachy velvety skin that's absolutely wasted on the young. She was an even-tempered, smiley baby who loved to lie on her back in a little patch of sunlight by the French doors in the family room. She was also content to go anywhere at any time, from car seat to plastic carrier to Snugli to sling.

My mother had never met my daughter. By the time Lizzie came along, my mother was well into her dementia. She did not know, she did not remember, that she had a new grandchild. Or, for that matter, that she had a daughter. When I took Lizzie with me for a visit two weeks after my mother had settled in, I was acutely aware of being a walking cliché, a poster child for the "sandwich generation." On one side of me I had a baby in diapers, on the other, a mommy in diapers. My daughter was learning as my mother was forgetting; my daughter was at the beginning, my mother was at the end. The symmetry was simultaneously startling and trite. I could imagine an essay on the subject. I could not imagine writing it.

My mother lived in one of five stand-alone, ranch-style houses, each with eight residents. That's how her Alzheimer's facility was set up. Each house actually *was* a house, with its own living room, dining room, and kitchen. The idea, of course, was to mimic a real home, which was achieved with somewhat limited success. Her house always seemed to be suffused with that cloying chemical fruit smell of plug-in bathroom deodorizers with a base note of Lysol. The furniture was all washable vinyl. The framed pictures on the walls were the kind bought by the dozen, sold by size and color. In my mother's room I had hung one of her own pictures, a pastel of a ballet dancer she had drawn while an art student at Pratt.

Whatever its shortcomings, the house was clean and bright, well staffed, and not nearly as institutional as the nursing homes and assisted-care facilities I had looked at. Three of the women in my mother's house were doll mothers. After my initial shock, I had begun to adjust to seeing them sitting shoulder to shoulder on the vinyl couch hugging and rocking their plastic babies. Knowing that I would soon be bringing a real baby into their midst, I wondered how they would react.

When Lizzie and I arrived that first day, the women were in their usual spots on the living room couch. I walked over and admired their babies, as I was now in the habit of doing, making those isn't-she-adorable comments strangers always make when they see babies. "And here's *my* baby," I said, presenting Lizzie so they could see her. One of the women did not look up. The other two glanced at my daughter, nodded politely, smiled, and went back to the bundles on their laps. Lizzie was waving her arms and amusing herself by blowing spit bubbles. It seemed inconceivable to me that they would not notice a difference between my baby and theirs. But they didn't. So we sat there for a few minutes, me on a nearby Naugahyde chair, cooing to Lizzie, them on the couch cooing to their infants, all of us pretty happy.

My mother had been getting her thrice weekly shower while all this was going on. A few minutes later she walked slowly and hesitantly into the living room, her hair damp and curly, her outfit one that I remembered, a kind of pre-tennis ensemble with navy blue stretch pants and a white zip-front cardigan with navy stripes up the sleeves. My mother had always looked young for her age. She took care of herself in the way of middle-class women of her generation: She got her hair "done" weekly; she gave herself regular manicures (she had beautiful hands); she wore foundation and mascara and lipstick every time she left the house, even to go grocery shopping. She also moved well. Into her seventies, she had no arthritis, no osteoporosis, no humps, no aches and pains, nothing to slow her down. She had been a graceful swimmer when she was younger and had been a decent, if unenthusiastic, tennis player well into middle age.

This woman walking toward me looked more like my grandmother than my mother. In fact, my grandmother, who was healthy and in her nineties at the time, looked better. This woman walking toward me had an impassive mask of a face. Her eyes were rheumy, and she was on her way to being too skinny for her clothes. She walked as though she had marbles in her shoes. It seemed to me that she'd aged two years in the two weeks she'd been at the facility. In a way, I guess, it helped that she was beginning to look less and less like herself. It made it a little easier to deal with the fact that she was unrecognizable in other, deeper ways.

I watched my mother reach out to steady herself against the

wall as she wobbled into the living room. Then I got up from the chair and, holding Lizzie in the crook of one arm, I hugged my mother with the other. Her body was stiff and tense. She didn't lean into me. I was some stranger putting my arms around her. We sat at one of the two small dining room tables so that she could drink her mid-morning cup of coffee. During our halting walk from living room to dining room, she had not noticed Lizzie. Now that we were seated, I presented my daughter to my mother.

"Here she is," I said. I'm afraid my voice had that fake-happy nursing-home ring to it. I spoke too loudly, like she was hard of hearing, which she wasn't. "Here's your new grandchild." My mother looked. Then something happened to her face. It was startling because I wasn't sure her face could register emotion anymore. At least I had not seen it. But now, suddenly, her face changed. She looked annoyed, then disgusted, then angry.

"What *is* that thing?" she said. "Get that thing away from me." I pulled Lizzie back into my arms and held her against my chest.

What I knew about Alzheimer's back then wasn't much. I don't think I really wanted to know more than I absolutely had to. But I did know that Alzheimer's often removed or muffled inhibitions, and that thus free from constraint, a person might speak or act in a way that seemed inappropriate or even bizarre. When my mother reacted that way to my daughter, I felt she was revealing something long buried, something that had been layered over by civility and propriety. *What is that thing?* Could this annoyance, this distaste, this aversion, really be my mother's true feeling about babies? And not just babies, of course, but *my* baby. And not just my baby, but me, her first baby.

I sat there holding Lizzie a little too tightly, watching my mother lift a mug of lukewarm coffee to her lips in slow motion, watching her take the smallest of sips, watching her struggle to swallow, and I thought of all the stories I had been told through the years about my own babyhood: how I ruined my mother's figure, how I had colic and eczema, how I got on my hands and knees and rocked in my crib, propelling it across the bedroom floor and making so much noise that my parents were asked to leave their apartment, how I picked up pennies from the street and put them in my mouth, and then had to have my gums swabbed with Gentian Violet. Growing up listening to these tales, I had somehow missed how entirely negative they were.

Two days after discovering Ella in the bathroom, I learn from Brooke, the administrator, that Ella is dead. The family, Brooke says, is sad but also relieved. There could have been interventions at the hospital. Her life might have been prolonged. But they decided against that. I will never know if the fall precipitated her death or if she fell because she was sick and dying. There will be no autopsy.

The news is hard to take. Two days ago we were giving Ella a shower. She was alert. She spoke to us. I know to expect death here, but I didn't expect it so soon. And on my watch. I go into Old Frances's room to cry. I can't cry out in the neighborhood because Jane, Eloise, Marianne, and Dottie are all with-it enough to notice and be disturbed. They don't know Ella has died. They've been told she was moved to another facility, which, in a way, is true. So I escape to Old Frances, who wouldn't notice tears, who wouldn't notice if I walked in with green spiked hair.

I see from the doorway that Old Frances is lying in her bed on her back, covered by her soft pink-flowered comforter. She has the nicest bedding of all the residents, the softest flannel nighties. Her eyes are opened. I walk into the room and immediately notice that something has been scrawled in black felt-tip pen across the hospice sign taped to the wall by her bed. "No Longer

On Hospice," it says. Old Frances has pulled through somehow! She's back with us. I lean down over her bed, wrap my arms around her bony little back, and give her the biggest hug I think she can handle.

"That's so nice," she says.

It's the first time I've ever heard her speak.

7

I haven't seen Jasmine, my old training partner, for more than a week. We're both on day shift, but she's been working weekends—an assignment that my privileged position allows me to decline—and on the days we're both here, she's been in a neighborhood across the atrium, which doesn't connect or share a common space with my neighborhood. But today, Jasmine is in 4, which links to 3, my bailiwick, via a broad hallway at the rear of the building. The doors across from both our kitchenettes open to a shared outdoor patio. Today we'll see each other.

Jasmine has more spirit than most of the people who work here. For them, this job, or this kind of job, defines not just their past but their present and their future. Among the RAs now in their forties, most were mothers in their teens and are now grandmothers several times over. It's hard for me to relate to them as contemporaries. But even the young ones, the twenty-somethings, seem old to me, with careworn faces and resigned attitudes reinforced by the realities of their lives. But I relate to Jasmine. She is not just another already defeated twentysomething who became a mother at seventeen and is fully submerged in the tough life of the working poor. She's got a spark. She sees that unless she takes control now, in twenty years she'll be another Lena, chain-smoking and bitching on a ten-minute break from some going-nowhere minimum-wage job, still living in a cheap apartment, still behind on her bills. The only difference is, she'll be a grandmother then. She sees the path, and she wants off. Unlike most of the women here, she believes she can change her life. She believes in the future.

Today we work in parallel universes and grab—or create—any opportunity we can to interact, if only for a moment. It's odd how close we feel, an almost instant intimacy based on those few days we spent together, bonding as we did over our mutual lack of self-confidence and joint awe in the presence of Calm Guam Frances. We borrow things from each other's neighborhoods (napkins, packets of sugar, gloves, laundry soap) even when we don't need to, just to touch base. When my residents are finished with lunch, and all the dishes are stacked on the cart, I push it through her neighborhood on the way to the kitchen, although it's more direct to go another way. When she sees me out on the patio checking on two of my residents who are sunning themselves on a bench, she finds an excuse to come out too.

These stolen moments are too brief to waste on small talk. We get right down to it. I learn that she's working as many extra shifts as she can trying hard to get ahead of her bills. She's already worked a couple of doubles, back-to-back shifts that keep her in the neighborhood from 6:30 a.m. to 10:30 p.m. I learn that it took her four years to qualify for "Section 8." I thought Section 8 was what they called you if you went nuts in the army, and they wanted to get rid of you. But apparently, Section 8 is also a federal program that helps low-income people with housing costs. Jasmine pays 30 percent of her income for housing—she and her son live in a boxy little apartment with matted wall-to-wall carpeting and wafer-thin walls—and the government picks up whatever is in excess of that percentage. The government also helps with childcare, after a co-pay that seems small but is, I know from my own paycheck, equal to three days' salary after taxes. She gets food stamps too, but the more shifts she works, the more money she makes, the fewer food stamps she gets.

Jasmine doesn't see her seven-year-old son much and has had little opportunity to talk to the woman who has been caring for him. She's in knots about this. She tells me about her sister who might come up from California to live with her. The sister doesn't sound like such a great bet to me—an unemployed high school dropout—but my job as Jasmine's one and only middle-class friend is to talk about possibilities, to encourage dreams, to keep her thinking about a way out. Jasmine says she and her sister can work out a schedule where the sister watches her son during the day and gets a part-time nightshift job somewhere. Meanwhile, Jasmine will find part-time day work and fit in classes at a community college. She'll get her GED. She'll get a two-year degree. The dream is a college degree and a job that pays a living wage. Yes, I tell her, yes. Right now, at Maplewood, if Jasmine works a forty-hour week, she brings home about $225. Somehow, she needs to save enough money to pay for her sister's bus ticket and then finance a move to a bigger apartment in a bigger city, where Jasmine wants to get a fresh start.

All this information I get in minute-long bursts as we move in and out of each other's neighborhoods for the next few days. An unexpected benefit of these visits with Jasmine is that I am getting to know her residents. These are people I see most every day because my neighborhood, neighborhood 3, is the hub of the facility. The activity Susan has scheduled for that day—a visiting musician, an exercise class, the twice-weekly balloon ball game—takes place in the common area in 3, so residents from all neighborhoods congregate here. I am slowing learning their names. I greet them. I give them hugs or back pats or arm squeezes, whatever seems appropriate. Touching is a big thing at Maplewood. Susan says—and I believe—that the elderly, sick or healthy, crave human touch. I trade small talk with these visiting residents, but I rarely get to know them. With people in my own neighborhood, I can piece together their histories by looking at the pictures in their rooms, talking to their relatives when they visit, and reading the abbreviated résumés we keep on file, the answers to questions about their past that relatives have provided. My curiosity is unflagging. I want to know their stories. Now, during my forays into Jasmine's neighborhood, I try to do that with a few of her residents. She takes me on quick tours of their rooms. She shares what she knows about their pasts.

I've been particularly interested in Caroline and Jack, the couple who always sit next to each other at the balloon ball games in my neighborhood. People have friends here, buddies they sit with or seek out. But Caroline and Jack seem different. They seem like a real couple, an old married couple—but also an odd couple. Jack is alert and talkative, a take-charge guy; Caroline is ghostly and vacant eyed, a stage ahead of Jack in the progression of the disease.

Caroline, I discover, was one of the original Rockettes onstage at Radio City Music Hall. She was a Lucille Ball redhead back then, with a perfect oval face, a tiny waist, and the requisite shapely legs. She has a framed picture of herself from those days sitting on her bureau next to a stack of Depends. Back then, Caroline was married to a guy also named Jack, a skinny Italian guy, a Sinatra look-alike from the eight-by-ten glossy in Caroline's room. From the form the family filled out when Caroline was first placed here, I learn that Jack played trombone in the Vaughn Monroe Orchestra, a popular swing band in the Big Band era. A careful, between-the-lines reading of Caroline's file reveals that her husband Jack was a hail-fellow-well-met kind of guy, a partyer, a big drinker, a lot of laughs. Caroline and Jack were married for forty-five more or less eventful years. Jack died fifteen years ago. These days Caroline has another man in her life, another Jack, also Italian. This is the guy she sits next to at balloon ball.

This Jack is short and stocky, a fireplug kind of a guy, who appropriately enough, used to be a fire chief. When I race over to visit Jasmine, I see Caroline and Jack sitting side by side on a big couch in the living room holding hands and watching a Shirley Temple movie on TV. Every time I'm in that neighborhood, they are never far from one another. They eat together, Jack sometimes feeding Caroline. They take short walks together, Caroline leaning heavily on Jack's arm. They go on forays into the adjoining corridors. Over in neighborhood 3 during activity time, they listen to a piano concert sitting side by side. The next day, they suffer through a group sing-along together. Caroline doesn't sing because she's too out of it. Jack doesn't sing because, he tells me proudly, the only way he can carry a tune is in a knapsack. The following day they are back listening to Jim Kelly's Blast from the Past, a visiting act featuring a lively septuagenarian couple dressed in identical purple cowboy shirts. He, bald and portly, plays a mean pedal-steel guitar. She, a little heavy on the pancake makeup, has a surprisingly clear Patsy Cline–like voice.

Caroline mostly walks around in a fog, the only visible object being Jack. But this afternoon, Jim Kelly's music gets to her. She is sitting in her seat next to Jack, listening to the duo and rocking her narrow hips back and forth. At first I think she needs to go to the bathroom, but then I see she's keeping time with the beat. She struggles to stand up, grasping the arms of the chair, her bony forearms shaking a little as she holds up her weight. Jack helps. When Caroline gets her balance, she begins rocking her hips again and taking tiny steps, side to side.

I walk over to her. "You like to dance?" I ask, just to make conversation, not expecting an answer.

She looks right at me. "Well," she says, "dancing is my life." Jack beams. He doesn't often get to hear Caroline talk. Or make sense.

The other day I spent both of my ten-minute breaks in neighborhood 4 talking to Jack. I bring up the subject of Italian food because chicken Parmesan is on the menu for lunch that day. Jack loves Italian food. He tells me that his father owned an Italian restaurant and did all the cooking at home too.

"It's the best food in the world," I say.

"You got that right," he says, and grabs my hand. He tells me that his favorite dish is lasagna.

"Chocolate lasagna?" Caroline says. I am sitting on one side of Jack; she is on the other. She looks down at Jack's hand clasping mine, and I swear this sweet, vacant-eyed lady shoots me a dirty look.

"Chocolate lasagna?" Jack says, pondering this idea, giving it his full attention. Then, a long minute later, he gets that it makes no sense, and he laughs and squeezes Caroline's hand.

I watch the two of them every chance I get. When I miss something, Jasmine gives me a report. They move together from couch to chairs back to couch again. Jack pats Caroline's cheek. Caroline strokes the top of Jack's head. They lean toward each other and touch dry lips. When Caroline has to go to the bathroom, Jack walks her there and waits outside the closed door.

When Jack goes to his room to look for something, Caroline follows him in, prompting Jasmine to make a dash for them. Caroline and Jack alone in a room may do something more than touch and kiss. I'm not sure if sex among Maplewoodians is expressly *verboten*. After all, these people are adults. But whether, in their altered states, they are *consenting* adults is another question—the same question, really, that faces those who run group homes for the mentally handicapped. I understand that here the relatives of the female residents for whom sex might be an issue are extremely protective. Caroline, even if she doesn't want to be, must be protected from her own libido as well as from the advances of Jack. The point is, I guess, that Caroline thinks this Jack is her old Jack, her husband.

What Jack thinks nobody really knows. He lost his wife seventeen years ago. She suffered a heart attack at home, and Jack, who knew CPR as well as any medic, Jack, who had spent his life saving people, couldn't save her. I imagine that he lived that long moment over and over in his mind, that it haunted him until Alzheimer's at first blunted and then erased the memory. Now Jack no longer remembers the specifics of the life he used to live, but he remembers that he is a person who takes care of people. And so he takes care of Caroline. Doing this gives his days a focus. He is pleasant and helpful and sometimes even jovial, a very different man, I discover talking to Susan and some of the old-timers, than the one who came here seven months ago.

Jack's family had brought him to Maplewood around dinnertime. By 7:30, he was yelling, tossing chairs around the room, and picking fights.

"You can't keep me here," he screamed at Stephanie, then the caregiver in neighborhood 4, now long gone, when she tried to calm him that first evening. "This is a prison, and I'm going to get out." The anger came and went. By eleven o'clock Jack had worked himself up again, deciding that the best way to get out of this strange place, this prison, was to start a fire. And he was just the guy to do it. Stephanie, who had read his file and knew he'd been a fire chief, took the threat seriously. She ran to his room and searched through the closet and the dresser drawers. Nothing. Then she patted him down and found a book of matches in his pocket. Jack disappeared into his room and started bashing the big picture window with a chair. "It's safety glass," Stephanie told him. He gave up and went back to yelling. By five in the morning, he had worn himself out, and the night-shift caregiver got him to bed. For weeks, every night at 7:30, he got agitated and restless and combative. Then he and Caroline connected, and life at Maplewood began to make sense to him. He settled in.

But before he found Caroline, he had a brief fling with Marla. Men are rare creatures here at Maplewood. Women outnumber them by at least four to one, sometimes six or seven to one. And men as hardy as Jack—ambulatory, talkative, dynamic—are even rarer. Here, diminished and at the end of his life, a man might find himself more popular, more in demand than he was in his prime. So Jack made a bit of splash when he arrived, his presence duly noted by those women with-it enough to note such things. First there was Marla, a pretty woman with snow white hair and oversized glasses flecked with dandruff who had just recently been cast off by another resident, the only other man in neighborhood 4 at the time, a big, strapping guy named William.

I tell Jasmine that I'm starting to get confused with all these names, all these couplings and uncouplings. She laughs and says that what I'm getting is the abbreviated version of all this, that there are twists and turns and even more names and potentially amorous encounters that complicate the drama even more. For example, William, who had been head of his own engineering firm and had, in his almost eighty years, gone through four wives and far too many bottles of whiskey, developed an eye for Marla's next-door neighbor, whose name I asked Jasmine please not to tell me. William's shift of attention to this other woman left Marla available for Jack, the newcomer.

Back then, Marla could still carry on a conversation and had no trouble feeding herself. Now she is mostly silent, and the RAs have to cut up her food. Jack and Marla were an item for about a week. But Marla was not demonstrative enough for Jack, not dependent enough on him. That's what the RAs thought at the time. How Jack looked at it was that Marla was not much interested in holding hands.

When Jack dumped Marla for Caroline, Marla's best friend, Jeanette, was quick to console her. "You don't need him," she told Marla. They were sitting together on the couch in the living room as they do now and did then, every afternoon. Jeanette was cleaning the white-specked lenses of Marla's glasses, as she does four or five times a day. "You're better off without him," Jeanette told her. "You'll see."

Now, many months later, Marla sees Jack and Caroline nuzzling each other, and it doesn't bother her a bit. It doesn't register. She has forgotten that she and Jack were ever together. But Jack has not entirely lost his eye for Marla. Occasionally, when he finds himself sitting next to her on the couch, he will take Marla's hand in his. Jack's other hand is, of course, holding Caroline's. Sometimes the three of them will walk together, Jack in the middle, guiding the two women.

Officially, this is neighborhood 4, but Jasmine and I and the other RAs call it—with wonder and amusement and not a hint of condescension—"Maplewood 90210" or "The Old and the Restless."

8

Today I am determined to spend some time with one of my residents named Marianne, the tall, attractive, well-dressed woman who doesn't look as if she belongs here. She is alert and pays attention. Her face registers a full range of emotions. Her eyes, especially, are focused and direct, so different from Old Frances's milky gaze or Addie's vacant stare or Eloise's now-I'm-here-now-I'm-not expression. I have been wanting to get to know Marianne, but she is so independent, so completely competent that, like the well-behaved child in a roomful of troublemakers, she is taken for granted. I knock on her door in the morning, and fifteen minutes later she is out sitting at one of the dining room tables, immaculately dressed, carefully coiffed, and ready for her morning cup of coffee. When it's her day for a shower, I remind her, and she takes care of it. Mid-morning and mid-afternoon, when there's an activity going on in the common area, I tell her about it a few minutes ahead of time, and she decides for herself whether she wants to participate. Truth is, she is so easy that I sometimes forget about her in my headlong, eight-hour rush to meet everyone else's needs. But today, I *will* find the time to sit with her. I've been told by Susan, by Calm Guam Frances, and by several others that Marianne is one of the most interesting residents here.

First, however, I must accomplish my least favorite post-breakfast chore: toileting. I am trying to be quick and efficient but also careful and caring, which is as difficult as it sounds. But that's the key to doing this job well. And doing this job well matters to me more and more as I become increasingly attached to the people in my care. I do Addie first because she is the hardest. She is wheelchair-bound and cannot support herself, even for a second, by holding onto the grab bar by the toilet. I have to position myself behind her, keep her upright by wedging my body against hers, a kind of upright spooning, with my legs, my quads, supporting her weight. She is not one of the little frail ones. Addie weighs 140. I wrap one arm around her ribcage while I pull down her Depends with the other hand. Then I hold her under her arms and inch back to position her on the toilet. I know I should not be doing this alone. Addie is a two-person assist, but I don't stop to call for help from the Float. If my sharp-tongued colleague Cathy saw me tackle Addie alone, she'd tattle on me to Christine. But I'm betting most RAs do whatever they think they can do, even when they shouldn't be doing it. There are just too many chores and too little time to wait around for assistance. Besides, I might as well use all those muscles I've been toning in the weight room.

I wheel Addie back out to the common area and am about to rush off to toilet Old Frances when I see that something is wrong. Addie's eyes are opened wide. She looks startled, fearful, in distress. I can't tell which.

"What's the matter, Addie?" I ask. She rarely speaks. "Does it hurt somewhere? Are you hurt?" She is pulling rollers from her hair. She's had her hair shampooed this morning in the little on-site salon, and because Addie cannot stand to be under a hair dryer, she was sent back to the neighborhood with her hair damp and wrapped in twenty soft pink curlers. Maybe the curlers are pinching her. I carefully unravel Addie's hair and then gently massage her scalp with the pads of my fingers. But that's not what's wrong. Her hands are shaking. She is picking at her pants. Maybe she has to go to the bathroom again. I take her there, heft her out of her wheelchair once again and onto the toilet—I am sweating now—but she doesn't go. I bring her out to the common area. She is breathing rapidly, fidgeting, jerking her head around.

I don't often think of Addie or any of the people in my charge as babies, even though often the level of care they need is similar to an infant's. But right now I am thinking of Addie as a baby because at this moment I feel the same fear and frustration I felt as a young mother trying to figure out why my firstborn was in distress. He couldn't tell me, just as Addie can't. So I would go through all the possibilities, step by step. Hungry? Wet? Needs to be rocked? Addie isn't hungry—she's actually eaten most of her breakfast—and she isn't wet. What does she need? How can I help? I kneel down next to her chair, put my arm around her, place my cheek next to hers. I can't tell if there are tears in her eyes because her eyes are always rheumy.

"What's wrong, Addie?" I ask again. I am afraid she may be in significant physical pain. I can't remember if she suffers from other ailments. So many of the residents do—high blood pressure, emphysema, coronary artery disease, diabetes. Maybe she's about to go into a diabetic coma.

"Can you tell me where it hurts?" I ask again, my face close to hers. Her hand is in her lap, shaking. She pulls it up toward her stomach, and I think, *okay, indigestion*. But then her hand moves to her chest, where it rests for a long moment. And I think, *jeezus, a heart attack. What do I do?* But her hand moves on, shaking, until it comes to her forehead.

"Here," she says. Somehow I know she doesn't mean she has a headache. She means something is wrong in there, in her head, and she doesn't know what.

"I know," I say. "I know." I get her a cup of juice with a straw. What else can I do?

I must move on to Old Frances. If I don't she'll be sitting in wet diapers, or worse, and neither of us will be happy. But where is she? I look around the dining room and the common area and don't see her. Where can a ninety-eight-year-old de-mented woman in a wheelchair go? Maybe I wheeled her back to her room and forgot? I rush to her room. No, she's not there. I am in a panic. I check the log book to see if her daughter came by when I wasn't looking and signed her out for a drive. Nope.

Did Rose come in while I was in the bathroom with Addie and steal Frances away? Rose has already been in the neighbor-hood twice this morning. I had to roust her out of Hayes's bed, one of her favorite spots, and had to redirect her when she fol-lowed me into another resident's room. Rose could be pushing Old Frances around the facility right now, Old Frances's feet catching under the wheelchair, Rose oblivious, Old Frances keel-ing over. When you have a moment, it's easy to catastrophize in this place, which is, after all, a world of potential catastrophes. It's a good thing I rarely have the time. I rush out to the front desk and ask Patty if she's seen Frances. She hasn't.

I don't really want to call on the walkie to ask if anyone has seen her (in Maplewood-speak, I would say: "Anyone have a vi-sual on 131?") because I don't want anyone to know that I've lost her. I go back and check all fourteen rooms and seven bathrooms in my neighborhood. No Frances. I sprint over to the adjoining neighborhood to see if, somehow, she got over there. I scan the common area. No Old Frances. I am out of ideas. Then, just as I am about to publicly announce, via the walkie, that I can't find one of my residents, Patty comes into the neighborhood to tell me that Frances is at the hairdresser, where Addie was earlier this morning.

In the large central atrium, perhaps twenty feet from the administrative offices and a small meeting room, is a tiny hair salon overseen by a large, intimidating sixty-something woman named Nona who, with her shellacked helmet of dyed hair, is a walking advertisement for the services she provides. Most of the women get their hair done by Nona once a week. It's an outing, something different, and they generally enjoy it. It costs extra, but many families pay. I think it's more important for the daughters who visit to see their mothers dolled up like they used to be than it is for the mothers themselves, most of whom never look in the mirror anymore and even if they did would probably not know who it was staring back. We RAs love it when Nona does her stuff because it means we have to do fewer shampoos. It also means we can write down an "activity" in our activity log, which is good, because families like to see that their loved ones are engaged in activities.

The tonsorial outcomes are, however, variable. Many of the women no longer have thick heads of hair. Many of them, in fact, have locks so wispy that they don't quite cover their pale pink and often scaly scalps. This is not good for Nona, who strives to replicate the full-helmet look with every head she touches. And so she back combs and teases until she builds a kind of thin-walled structure around the scalp held up by the tensile strength of hair-spray. Frances is wheeled back a few minutes later, her hair teased to an inch of its life, her Depends, I can tell in an instant, full of poop. I don't care. I'm just thrilled to see her.

Finally, with a half hour until lunch, I have time for Marianne. I know from the questionnaire filled out by her brother, who brought her here four months ago, that she is a former university administrator, a college-educated career woman who married but never had children in an era—Marianne is seventy-eight—where that decision would have set her apart. This morning, Marianne is dressed in trim black slacks, a tailored ivory silk blouse, and a cropped Chanel jacket. She has a good leather purse slung over her shoulder and is sitting, back erect, legs crossed, hands clasped in her lap, in a chair just outside the door to her room. She looks ready to leave for a power lunch.

I walk over to say hello. The protocol, the etiquette, what we all do around here, is to greet a resident by patting an arm or rubbing a back. Touch is vital when dealing with folks who may have limited understanding of words. It feels natural and right to do this, warm without being too personal. But Marianne immediately inspires a handshake. I cannot imagine the intimacy of rubbing her back. It would be as unthinkable as a fifth grader greeting her principal by patting her on the arm.

"Hello," I say, not sure how to begin the conversation. Usually I will ask, "How are you feeling today?" or "Are you having a good day?" but that seems, like the back rubbing, too casual, as if I am presuming a certain kind of relationship which everything about Marianne tells me not to presume. "I was wondering if we could talk for a moment," I say, stalling. She gives me the subtlest of once-overs.

"Of course," she says. "Shall we go into my office?" Her *office*? She opens the door to her bedroom and ushers me in. I sit on one of the chairs. She chooses the bed, which I find a little odd, but then I see that sitting on the bed puts her in a higher position than me. She sets down her purse by her side, crosses her legs, and looks down at me. "Now, how can I help you today?" she asks politely.

This is awkward. Marianne is not some sweet-faced, hazy-minded old lady with whom I can exchange pleasantries about the pretty sweater she's wearing or the flowers blooming outside her window. I try to feel my way into the conversation. "I was hoping we could talk a little bit about your impressions of this place," I say, mirroring her formality.

"Of course," she says. "I will say first that this has been a very satisfying position for me. It's an open-ended sort of position you can make of what you want." She pauses and smiles faintly. "Within certain parameters, of course." She articulates every word, like someone who has taken elocution lessons. Her voice has that modulated, accentless tone of the well educated. She talks about the employees here. "I value what they do," she tells me, "but I often find their productivity is lacking." Marianne, it is gradually dawning on me, believes she is an administrator here at Maplewood. What kind of a place she thinks Maplewood is, I have yet to discover.

This woman goes against everything I thought I knew about Alzheimer's. I thought the disease stripped away the outer layers, the public layers, that over time if Alzheimer's left anything, it left the distilled essence of the person—Jack's sense that he is someone who helps people, Rose's restless soul. But Marianne's outer layers are very much intact. Or maybe I'm looking at it the wrong way. Perhaps this *is* Marianne's essence. After all, she spent a half century as a career woman, starting a job when most women, like my mother, were starting families in the new post-war suburbs. This is how she defined herself, and it's how she defines herself now. So maybe it makes sense that this part of Marianne remains untouched by brain plaques and nerve tangles.

I can't help thinking how wonderfully enriching and protective this world is that she has decided to live in. It gives her a reason to get up in the morning, a reason to dress meticulously. It shields her from the knowledge that she is ill and spends every day around other people who are ill. It shields her from the knowledge that she is alone. I love that Marianne's brain works this way. I like to think that it is paying her back for all the years she used her mind so well, the years she cared for it by thinking and reading and organizing and planning, stimulating it, stuffing it with information, creating pathways, bridging synapses. It was a well-used brain, and now it's working on autopilot.

We talk for twenty minutes in her "office." I feel compelled to stay completely within her reality, to ask what would be appropriate questions and respond in appropriate ways if she actually were an administrator here. As we talk, I don't feel that I am playing a game. What I'm doing doesn't feel like a trick. It is a matter of respecting Marianne and who she is. If I were her daughter—if she had a daughter—I'd be completed freaked out. Marianne's delusions would seem weird and disturbing. I'd probably cry after every visit. But as her caregiver, as a person who never knew the "real" Marianne, I am fascinated.

"Why exactly have you come to see me?" she asks at one point. I hesitate, look down, try to think fast. I can't tell her that I want to talk to her about life in the care facility because whatever she thinks Maplewood is, she doesn't think it's an Alzheimer's home. I can't tell her the truth about why we're talking, about who I am and where we are, so I say, simply, that I heard from the top administrator here that Marianne was a good person to talk to, which is absolutely true.

"I hope we can talk again later," I say. "I will be around quite a lot." She considers this.

"My schedule is somewhat busy," she tells me. "I am not sure when I will be available."

"It would be best to set up an appointment in advance, then?" I ask. I hear myself say this and realize that I am not at all pretending. Marianne has roped me into her reality. She asks for my business card. I hand it to her, shake her hand, and walk out the door.

The way I am with Marianne is partly instinctive—it just feels right—and partly a result of the reading I've been doing on something called validation therapy, a novel approach to dealing with people who suffer from memory loss. Not too long ago, the standard approach taken by health professionals was known as "reality orientation," which involved constantly correcting those with Alzheimer's in an effort to keep them grounded in the actual and factual. So, if a demented person started talking about the lunch she just had with her mother, a woman who was actually long dead, the response might be: "This is 2006. Your mother died thirty years ago. The person you had lunch with was your daughter." The idea was that by keeping a person connected to the real world you could postpone total confusion.

Not knowing this approach was called anything, or that it was in disrepute, or that there *was* another approach, I relentlessly practiced reality orientation with my mother. I always corrected her when she called me Judy (her sister). Every time I visited, I took down the framed photographs from her dresser—the ones I had brought in to remind her of her family—pointed to each, and quizzed her. "You know who this is, don't you, Mom?"

Of course, she didn't. So I told her, again and again, each visit, who was who. And then quizzed again. When she would not step across a crack in the sidewalk, seeing it, I now know, as a shadowy gulf, I pooh-poohed her fear. "It's nothing. Just a line in the concrete. *Come on, Mom.*" Thinking back on this now, I am appalled at my insensitivity. What did I think I was doing? After months of reality orientation, I managed to accomplish only two things: I made myself miserable, and I made my mother irritable. I see relatives do this every day at Maplewood—disagree, contradict, correct, challenge.

I know they mean well, just as I meant well. I know they think they're helping. But they're not. They are actually doing harm. A Cleveland social worker by the name of Naomi Feil noticed that repeatedly correcting those with Alzheimer's made them withdrawn or hostile. Not surprisingly, they sometimes became combative—no one likes to be contradicted all the time—or paranoid—*why is everyone always saying I'm wrong?*—or simply stressed. I notice this stress response here in the neighborhood after relatives leave.

Suppose, Feil thought, caregivers (family members or professionals) adjusted to the person with Alzheimer's rather than trying to force the person to adjust to them? Suppose caregivers tuned in to the reality being lived by the person with Alzheimer's rather than trying to force another reality upon them? Feil's approach, called validation therapy, is based on respect for the end-of-life process. She believes that the elderly—those both with and without memory problems—want and need to return to their past as a way of resolving life issues before they die. She sees living in the past not as a symptom of brain disease but rather as a survival technique. An older person returns to the past to relive the good times and deal with the bad as a way of wrapping up loose ends, a way of coming to closure and finding peace.

And so, you go where that person is going. You don't challenge or contradict or correct. You listen. You respond in a way that encourages conversation. Feil's validation therapy is practical, sensitive, intuitive—and mind-bending. When you practice it, you are not only keeping stress levels down and opening channels of communication. You are not only respecting the dignity of the other person. You are actually being forced to consider that a person with Alzheimer's might be doing important life work right in front of you.

A few days later, Marianne catches me mid-morning. Today she is dressed in tan slacks, a taupe blouse, and a short, boxy jacket, her leather purse, as always, hanging from her shoulder. I've been sitting with Eloise and Jane, jumping up periodically to change the laundry, excusing myself to check on Hayes, to put in a new video (a stunning travel documentary of New Zealand—there is just so much Lawrence Welk a person can take), to pour cups of juice for those who hang out around the dining room tables between meals.

"Can you tell me when luncheon will be served?" Marianne asks me.

"Twelve thirty," I tell her, "about two hours from now."

"And do you know what might be on the menu?"

"I think I can smell it," I say. "It's meatloaf." I get up to check the menu posted on the wall of the kitchenette. "Yep, meatloaf. There's also scalloped potatoes and green beans and applesauce."

"My, my," says Marianne, moving back to take a seat by the door to her room. She places her purse on her lap.

"Can you tell me when luncheon might be served?" Marianne

is out of her chair walking toward the kitchen again. It's been no more than three minutes since she last asked the question. I tell her again, then enumerate the menu items. Marianne nods and thanks me as she walks back to her chair. A minute later, she is back again.

"Can you tell me when luncheon might be served?" She repeats herself perfectly. Her inflection is identical. She has that same look of detached, mild curiosity. I am seeing short-term memory loss at its most extreme, and it is very hard to watch. I like to think of Marianne as perfectly fine within her own world, as a fully functioning person. As she listens to my response for the third time, I can see that all of a sudden she realizes she is hearing information she has heard before. She loses that detached look and shakes her head. "My mind seems to be a sieve," she says. No self-pity, no criticism, no apology, just an honest assessment, like an administrator evaluating a worker.

While we wait for lunch, Marianne agrees to talk with me again.

"Yes," she says, "I do have some time now."

I ask her for her impressions of "this place," careful to be vague, not knowing what she calls Maplewood in her head. From our conversation the other day, I have no idea what she thinks Maplewood is, but she made it quite clear, I thought, that she believes she holds an administrative post here. So it takes me by surprise when she says, "This place is wonderful. It gives us a place to relax, we women who are so busy with our careers. We need a place like this."

She goes on to describe what sounds like a corporate retreat for female executives. Then she launches into one of the most articulate, informed discussions of the successes of the feminist movement that I've ever heard. She talks about "matriculating as a person" and "graduating into a state of mind of equality." Her language is as eloquent as her thinking. She talks about her husband learning to "become unaccustomed to the dominant role he presumed from birth." She talks about women learning to present themselves in the world. This is a woman who graduated from college in 1948, a woman who figured out how to be a feminist while Betty Friedan was still working it out. Does it matter, really, that she forgets when lunch will be served?

9

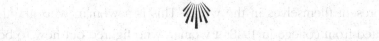

One day after work, sweating and panting my way through a late-afternoon workout at the athletic club, I find myself on an EFX machine next to Gail, a lockerroom acquaintance. She asks me how my summer is going, expecting, I am sure, the usual *just great . . . and what've you been up to?* but getting instead an earful about Maplewood. I guess I need to talk. I tell her how physically demanding the work is, how I am always in motion, hefting, bending, lifting. I tell her about how, during my first weeks on the job, I would come home mid-afternoon and pass out on the couch until dinnertime, which concerned my husband—and not just because it meant he had to make dinner every night. I was the one with a deep, seemingly inexhaustible well of energy. In the many years we had been together, he had never seen me take a nap. I start telling Gail about Ella—I have not made peace with her death and what part I might have played in it—but I choke up and can't get through the story. Gail looks over at me, worried. I feel the need, immediately, to explain, defend, set her straight. "But I *love* this job," I tell her. "I truly love it." Now she *really* looks worried.

It's hard to explain. And it has taken me by surprise. But it's true: I do love the job. I have cared about doing it well from the start—both as a matter of personal pride and an homage-apologia to my mother. But it is more than that now. As tired as I am when my shift is done, I look forward to work the next day. When I'm not there for a few days, I miss the place. I miss Jasmine and Calm Guam Frances and Angela, a new easygoing, soft-spoken Med Aide. I miss perennially perky Susan and salt-of-the-earth Patty at the reception desk and even Nona, the helmet-headed hairdresser. But mostly I miss the residents. They are, collectively and individually, a handful, but they are also endearing and, in their own ways, spirited. I enjoy their company. Their dementias and delusions, their personalities, are fascinating and distinct. Figuring out who they are and what makes them tick is intellectually and emotionally challenging. It is also deeply satisfying.

When I tell Gail or my friends or my husband that I love this work, they don't get it. They know about my mother and the emotional baggage I carry with me to work every day. And they think they know about Alzheimer's—that is, they know the dark, depressing stuff they read in the media. So how can I enjoy spending time with demented people? How can I like my job? How can I, in fact, *stand* my job? Susan tells me she has the same problem explaining her work to others. She says that telling people she works with Alzheimer's patients is a real conversation stopper.

Hayes is everything that is both exhausting and exhilarating about this job. Of all the people in the neighborhood, he easily wins the award for Highest Maintenance Resident. If awake, he demands attention. If he's out of his room, you better be there right next to him or he'll make sure you regret it. He is forever yelling. He needs help with absolutely everything. Yet the man is, somehow, a charmer. Just when you want to throttle him (I don't mean literally, of course, so eldercare advocates, *please stand down*), he pats your hand and thanks you. Just when you have exhausted the very last smidgen of patience, he delivers a witty line. When you're sure he doesn't understand, he says something so insightful it takes your breath away. Then, that neatly accomplished, he goes back to being a bossy, cranky, difficult old coot.

Whenever I wheel him from one place to another or minister to him in any way, he always asks, "What's next? What's next?" He wants to know, step by very small step, what is happening, where we're going, what we're doing, what is expected of him. I can't just say, "Hayes, now we're going to brush your teeth." He wants it broken down. He wants me to tell him that now I am putting the toothpaste on the brush and now he is to open his mouth and now I am brushing the top teeth and now he should spit and yes, he can spit again. This is beginning to drive me crazy.

This morning I get him to grab his walker and pull himself up out of his chair, but I can't just say, "Let's go to breakfast," because once Hayes is standing, he will freeze and ask, "What's next?" So I say, "We are going to walk over to your wheelchair," which is not good enough, because he advances one or two steps, then stops and asks, "What's next?" I have to say, "Now we are walking a few more steps." And "Now we are almost there." And "Now you are going to sit in the wheelchair." The process of sitting has many steps, all of which I must delineate out loud for Hayes: take two steps back (*what's next?*), shift your hands (first right, then left) from the walker to the arms of the chair (*what's next?*), bend your knees, lower yourself down (*what's next?*), sit back, move your legs (first right, then left) onto the leg supports (*what's next?*). I am getting hoarse.

I am also getting impatient. Isn't it enough that I do all this for him . . . I have to keep up a running commentary too? It's annoying. It slows everything. It keeps me from other tasks. As I go through the motions this morning, detailing the minutiae of Hayes's life for him, I think about the man. I have read all the material we have on Hayes. I know that he grew up on the prairie outside of Alberta, Canada. I know he went to a one-room schoolhouse and was taught by his aunt. I know his wife is named Mabel. I remember that he was a mechanical engineer by trade.

Then it starts to make sense: the way he has to know every detail, the way he wants every process broken down into small steps, the way he can't move until he knows what's next. This must be how he lived his occupational life. This must be how he sees the world. This must be how his brain works. Although other parts of his brain may not be working very well, this step-by-step detail part sure does. The second I make that connection, my impatience disappears, and I begin to admire how orderly and logical Hayes is, how much of his essence is still intact. It also gives me a positive way of interacting with him. I will no longer wait for him to ask, "What's next?" because by the time he says it, he is already beginning to feel anxious. There is already agitation in his voice. I will talk him through everything we do as we are doing it. I will treat him like the methodical, systematic, organized engineer he was.

I try this during the morning routines, and it's stunning how well it works. Hayes is cooperative and calm. He seems happier. His demands are less frequent and less strident. I sit him down on his big chair by the window and tell him I'm going to walk over and put some music on his CD player. As I look through his collection—Sinatra, Jolson, the Dorsey brothers, Glenn Miller—Hayes starts to sing "You're in the army now / You're not behind a plow." I know that ditty. My father, who fought in World War II, used to sing it sometimes. I sing along in my head: "You'll never get rich by diggin' a ditch / You're in the army now."

When he finishes singing, Hayes segues into a spontaneous monologue about how he never wanted to go into the army. No, no, the army was not for him. And I wonder what exactly he's talking about. He would have been six years old when the Great War was being fought and almost thirty and married with four or five of his nine children already born by the time America entered World War II. Did the army want him then?

There's a lot of history locked up inside this man's head. Alzheimer's locked it in, but even without the disease, even if all those memories were accessible, I wonder who would take the time to listen. Are there really cultures that listen to, even revere, their elders? I know I've read about them—American Indians, the Chinese—but they seem impossibly remote, almost mythological. What I see, what I've experienced, is old people, healthy and sick, living solitary, silent lives; old people made to feel as if they need to apologize for being old, for clogging up the works, for showing us the future we don't want to see. So we lose patience when standing behind a grandma at the grocery store. She's fiddling with coupons. She's taking forever to count out the change from her purse. *Come on.* The geezer in the car, who actually makes a full stop at the stop sign and looks both ways before proceeding. The grandpa who pulls out the old photo album. We roll our eyes and find the first excuse to leave the room.

Later, in the bathroom, Hayes is fussing. It is taking me too long to get his three layers of bottoms—briefs, long johns, khakis—up and adjusted. It's difficult to zip his fly and button the button with my latex gloves on.

"Take me out, take me out," he yells at me as I kneel in front of him fiddling with his pants. I try to calm him, tell him I'm working as fast as I can, tell him what steps I'm taking. But he's agitated now. "Take me out. Take me out." He's mad. I get flustered and zip the index finger of my glove into his fly. "Take me out." He's really yelling now. I need help, but I'm not going to get it. "Take me out!" he yells again, and for some reason, I hear it differently this time, and I start to sing, "Take me out to the ball game." I've heard Hayes sing this song. "Take me out to the ball game / Take me out with the crowd," I sing loudly. And poorly. I rarely sing in public. But here I am singing in Hayes's bathroom while I extricate the finger of my glove from his fly. Before the first verse is finished, he is singing along. I don't know all the words, but he does.

With an hour before lunch, Hayes nodding off in his chair, I turn my attention to Eloise, who needs a shower. This shouldn't be a problem—Eloise is one of my favorites; we have a rapport—but it *is* a problem. Eloise is making a fuss. The water is too cold. The water is too hot. My hands are too cold. *Don't do that. Don't touch me. Ouch!* She flinches as if being stung when I direct a gentle spray of water on her feet. She is sitting naked on a plastic bench set in the big walk-in shower in her bathroom. I am standing next to her holding the spray nozzle in one hand, stroking her back with the other.

When I started working here I was astonished at the residents' lack of modesty. My job requires me to be intimate with them. I see everyone naked. I touch flesh. I heft breasts into bras. I wash private parts. I blot vaginas and wipe butts. I was, at first, embarrassed by this intimacy, but I saw very quickly that *they* weren't—

which freed me not to be. With some of the residents this lack of modesty is part of a general lack of awareness, the brain-disease trance they're in. But with others, like Eloise, I think it comes from a different place. I think it's an almost saintly acknowledgment of their own vulnerability, a calm, open acceptance of their own needs and the fact that now others must be involved in helping them. It's Eloise's lack of vanity, her peaceful, artless humility that makes it possible for me to do what I do. It's really, when I think of it, a gift Eloise and the others give me—although right now, standing in the shower with Eloise, it doesn't feel like much of a gift. My sneakers are soaked. I'm sweating. It's taken us almost fifteen minutes to get to this point. *That's cold,* she yells when the water cascades down her back. Eloise never yells. I check the temperature again. It's comfortably warm.

I've seen these over-the-top visceral reactions with others, not just about water, not just about temperature, but about anything that touches them—a warm breeze, a shawl, my hands. Hayes can't stand anything rough against his skin. He will yell *ouch!* when his arm slides in the sleeve of a soft flannel shirt. He will complain about the feel of fluffy, warm-from-the-dryer cotton socks on his feet. I'm struggling to understand. Later I ask a doctor I know, the father of one of my daughter's school friends who also happens to be the medical director of the local hospital's eldercare unit. I tell him about my theory that people with Alzheimer's compensate for their cognitive fuzziness with an overly acute tactile sense. He thinks I might be right about the heightening of certain senses, but he doesn't really know. It's astonishing what we don't know about the experience of having Alzheimer's, he tells me. We pay more attention to the death of a neuron than to the life of the person. I know the medical approach is vital. We've got to discover what causes Alzheimer's. We've got to find a cure. But caring for my residents, and thinking about the four and a half million others living with this disease, I wish we spent more research dollars on exploring and trying to understand the realities of their lives.

Eloise objects all through the shower. She's not just grouchy; she's angry, almost combative. With all my coaxing, with all the goodwill I've racked up with Eloise during the past month—we exchange at least a dozen hugs a day—I can barely get her to tolerate a soft stream of water on her back. I give up on the idea of a shampoo, although she sorely needs one. I finish the shower as quickly as I can, wrap her in two dry towels, and get her seated on the toilet. This is the easiest position from which to get her dressed.

I kneel in front of her, pull her Depends up to just above her knees, then struggle with the impossibly tight medical support hose she wears for edema, then pull her pants to mid-thigh. That way when she stands I can get everything positioned quickly and at once. She looks down at me as I slip her foot into a shoe, and with one hand sweeps the wisps of hair away from my sweaty face. It's a mother's touch.

"Don't you ever get tired of taking care of us old bags?" she asks me sweetly. These are the first words she's said to me in an hour that sound like the Eloise I've come to know. I have to laugh.

"I'll be an old bag some day myself," I tell her.

At lunch out in the workers' al fresco breakroom—the poured concrete slab nestled between the back of the building and the garbage cans—I sit at the plastic picnic table upwind from Lena, who is, as usual, chain-smoking. In between deep drags, she is giving me an earful about how her son or maybe son-in-law is moving back in and how she's taking care of two of her grandchildren who were abandoned by her daughter who lives in

California with a crack dealer and how her husband is a lazy bum and how she had to work eleven hours yesterday because swing shift didn't show up. I listen and realize that Lena's reality, her chaotic nickel-and-dimed world, is far more unreal to me than any of Marianne's delusions.

It's lunch break, but Lena is not eating. "You ought to get something," I tell her. I'm not really thinking about her nutrition; I'm thinking that if her mouth is full she will stop talking.

"I got something out of the machine," she tells me. That means, at best, a bag of Doritos. I ask her how, if she doesn't eat lunch, she keeps up her strength for working. She's forty-five but looks like a hard sixty.

She shrugs. "I guess I feed my kids better than I feed myself," she says. She means her grandkids. She tells me that last night she went out and got them macaroni and cheese and chicken strips. She smokes and watches me eat the salad I brought from home.

"I bought fresh vegetables once," she says. I nod encouragingly. She takes another drag. "They stayed in the refrigerator until they rotted."

After Lena, it's a relief to get back to the neighborhood. The afternoon goes well. Hayes is responding to my new strategy. I've weathered tropical storm Eloise, and she's back to being her sweet self. I manage to give another resident, Pam, the one attached to the oxygen tank, a shower when no one—not even Calm Guam Frances, who was working this neighborhood yesterday—could do it. I've got something good going with Marianne. There are moments, long moments, when what was frantic activity becomes fluid motion, when I move from task to task with not just efficiency but a kind of grace. I am busy, but I am not frenzied. I find a rhythm. I work up a sweat. I am in the zone.

The only downer is Rose. I trail after her all afternoon. She is taking socks from Addie's dresser. She is lying in a fetal position on Hayes's bed. She is in May's room about to "borrow" one of her photographs. She is in the little kitchen reaching for a cup of hot coffee I've just poured for Eloise. She is walking away with a pile of Old Frances's clean laundry that I left stacked on a chair.

She is everywhere, shuffling, blank eyed, impassive. I look at her walking away, noting the sag of her wet diaper under her polyester pull-on pants, and I wonder how far this woman walks in a day. I wonder where all this energy comes from, this force that keeps her moving, keeps her restless and uncomfortable in her body and in this place. I take her arm and walk her out of the neighborhood. Of course she is back in less than two minutes. I call over to the RA in her neighborhood, and ask for someone to come over and get her. Someone does, but Rose is back again in ten minutes, this time clutching a cookie in her hand.

I am busy tending to Addie. When I track down Rose a few minutes later, I am too late. She has smeared her greasy, cookie-crumb hands all over Hayes's pillowcase and comforter. I will have to strip his bed, remake it, and do a separate load of wash. Hayes's linens must be washed only in the special laundry soap brought by one of his daughters. I try to move Rose off the bed, but she won't budge. She pulls her arm out of my gentle grasp and gives me a look I can't describe. There is little intelligence behind the look, so I can't say it is a look of hatred or annoyance, or that there is anything actually definable in the look. But I can tell you it's scary. I try to push away the thought, but I can't: Rose is a zombie—a body that lives without a brain, a body that lives without a soul.

Once I get her out of the neighborhood, with the help of both Susan and the Float, I breathe easier. I get a hug from Eloise. I pour Marianne a fresh cup of decaf. I kid around with Jane. I find my rhythm again.

I am, I tell myself, at the top of my game. I figure it's only a matter of time until I see my name on one of the yellow construction paper stars thumbtacked to the employee bulletin board. Anyone who works here can fill out a star in praise of any other worker. *Awesome job, Kim. Cynthia . . . You rock.* It's really a lame attempt at morale building that costs this place nothing—unlike, say, *a raise* for doing extraordinary work—but it gives the appearance of "staff appreciation." I am thinking that some corporate boss or HR bureaucrat heard about this star thing at an employee-relations seminar. There's a whiff of kindergarten about it too.

Given my cynicism, it comes as a shock to me when I realize, at the end of my shift as I look at the sprinkling of stars on the board, that *I want a star!* I want my name up there. I want the great job that I think I'm doing publicly recognized. I fleetingly consider making a secret deal with Jasmine: If she'll scrawl *Lauren's the best* on a star, I'll write *We love Jasmine* on another. But that's cheating. I want an honest star. No. What I really want is what I can't have, what I blew my chances for: I want a star for taking care of my mother. I want a star for being a good daughter.

10

On my next day off, I arrange to visit Hayes's daughter Jennie, one of his nine children, the one most involved in his life right now. I rarely see Jennie at Maplewood—her frequent visits don't coincide with my work schedule—but I have noticed her hand everywhere: in the blue plaid flannel sheets she buys for him, in his wardrobe of Gap sports shirts and crisp khakis, in the little ziplocked bags of premeasured Ivory Snow she sets on his closet shelf. Maplewood's industrial-strength detergent irritates Hayes's sensitive skin. Jennie pays attention to things like that, to the little details of her father's life.

I think about Jennie every time I go to dress Hayes. With some of the other residents, I have to paw through drawers filled with torn underwear, mismatched socks, hookless bras, and permanently stained shirts to find something decent for them to wear. Their relatives, even if they care—which many of them do—even if they come to visit regularly, seem to miss this detail. Maybe they are overwhelmed with the reality of the disease; maybe they are too busy with their own lives. Or maybe they think it doesn't matter what dad or grandma wears. Maplewood is an institution, after all, not the outside world. The only people who will see dad or grandma are other old folks with Alzheimer's, paid caregivers, and family.

But I think it does matter. It matters to some of the residents, even the ones you might think are too out of it to know what they are wearing. I remember the huge smile on Old Frances's face when I put a new, soft flannel nightgown over her head. "Nice," she said. It was the only word she said that day. And the clothes matter to me. It is a pleasure to dress someone in attractive clothing, to see Hayes looking spiffy or Eloise, elegant. It helps me think of them as people, not patients. It boosts my morale just by looking at them, and maybe, although I don't want to admit this, it causes me to treat them a little differently, with a little more respect. It certainly shows me that the family treats them with respect, that the family sees the person and not just the disease. It shows me that the family has not given up.

That's the thing about Hayes's daughter Jennie: She hasn't given up. The time and effort and attention she devotes to her father's life shows in his clothing—no missing buttons, no frayed cuffs, no stains, new pajamas that appear when the elastic waistbands of old ones grow weary, a drawer full of brilliant white socks. She makes it easy for us caregivers to keep Hayes looking good. One of my co-workers complains about the special Ivory Snow treatment we're supposed to give Hayes's laundry—just one more thing to remember in the midst of a hectic day—but the rest of us think it's wonderful. His clothes smell nicer than anyone else's, and they feel softer. Jennie has also taped neatly hand-printed labels on all of Hayes's dresser drawers: underwear and longjohns, reads one; collared shirts and sweaters, reads another. It's a small thing, but in my world of running from resident to resident, from chore to chore, the labels are a blessing. Putting away Hayes's clean laundry is easy. Finding the right clothes is quick. I silently thank Jennie every day. I want to know her secret, the secret to not giving up.

And so, I call her and arrange a visit. She and her second husband live twenty minutes from Maplewood. Their home is a modest cottage on a quiet street. To reach the front door, I walk through an arched trellis into a small brick courtyard and through a pocket garden. The effect is immediately, powerfully welcoming. Inside, the house is immaculate but homey. Everything is organized but not fussy. Jennie is like her house: small, pretty, and unaffected. She has the trim figure of a twenty-five-year-old and a soft, comely face that shows both her age and her comfort with it. She is sixty-six, Hayes's second-oldest child.

I want to know all about Hayes, I tell her. Really, I want to know all about her, but I think I can best get to this by listening to what she says about her father. It's clear she wants to talk. I barely have to pose a question. When I listen, I am at first so struck by *how* she speaks about her father that I don't pay much attention to *what* she says. She isn't sad, her voice doesn't crack with emotion, she doesn't look away. She isn't angry or regretful or even wistful. This is so different from conversations I've had at Maplewood with other residents' family members. Just as I was when people used to ask me about my mother, they seem either incurably melancholic or deeply uncomfortable or both. But Jennie is enjoying talking about her father. And it's not because she is choosing to tell me some Norman Rockwell version of his life.

She tells me that Hayes, at age eight, was waking before dawn to do chores and then hitch up the horse and buggy to drive himself and four younger siblings to school. His father was tough on him, she says, and favored his younger, smarter brother. This she found out not from Hayes himself—"My father rarely spoke," she says, shaking her head, "I mean *rarely*"—but from an aunt.

We kids respected him, she tells me, but we didn't know him. He was kind but remote, a physical presence but not an emotional one. Jennie was already married and herself a mother, she says, when Hayes and his wife, Mabel, had their ninth and final child. The boy was two when Hayes left him alone in his machine shop for a few minutes. The child climbed up on a shelf and managed to dislodge a heavy object that crashed down on him and crushed him to death. Jennie's voice is now just above a whisper. The real tragedy, she says, was that Hayes never spoke of the accident. And so the family never spoke of it. Instead, her father went deeper into himself than ever, became even more distant, even more silent.

Alzheimer's changed all that. If there's one thing Hayes is not, it is silent. He is the least silent person in the neighborhood. The literature of the disease speaks of "personality change" but always in the negative: the docile old lady who starts cursing and biting; the previously perfect husband who throws a chair at his wife; the prim grandma who all of a sudden likes to walk around naked. When these changes happen to people with Alzheimer's, as they in fact do, family members are appalled and embarrassed. But really these new "behaviors," as they are called in the Alzheimer's care community, are not weird, disease-induced metamorphoses but a kind of transparency. The behaviors, or the impetus for them, were probably always there, always part of the personality, but they were repressed or ignored or paved over by a veneer of what was acceptable or expected, what was encouraged and rewarded. Jung called this hidden side of us the "shadow self." And so maybe the prim grandma had a sexual side she was never able to express that the disease now, much to the family's consternation, "liberates." Or it may be that the well-behaved husband tamped down anger and frustration for decades but is now, under the influence of Alzheimer's, suddenly free to express it.

All this helps explain Hayes. As I listen to Jennie talk about her stolid and stoic father, I think: That's what a man was supposed to be, especially a man who came of age during the Great Depression, especially a man at the helm of a family of ten, especially a man made to feel, early on, as if he were not good enough. But Hayes must have also had a part of him that wanted to speak up, that wanted to say: *I'm Hayes. Pay attention to me. I need things too,* a part that wanted to talk and talk and maybe even sing and show the world he existed. While he was busy being the strong, silent type, he must have harbored, as we all harbor, a part of himself that was needy and vulnerable. What Alzheimer's did was clear the way for all this to come through.

Now Hayes is letting it all out. He is talkative and demanding. He complains. He yells at you if you bump his wheelchair against a door frame, if you try to pull his arm through the sleeve of his shirt, if you leave his side for a moment during mealtime. He craves—and loudly insists on—the attention he never got. Hayes is a very difficult man.

But that is not how Jennie thinks of him, and maybe that's why she's been able to be such a good daughter. Jennie is not a head-in-the-clouds woman. She taught elementary school for three decades, went through a tough first marriage, raised her kids mostly on her own. She's clear-eyed and matter-of-fact, warm but also disciplined and no-nonsense. She is the kind of woman who puts labels on dresser drawers. That's why it comes as a surprise when Jennie tells me that she sees Alzheimer's as a gift. *Gift* is the word she uses. I have heard people call cancer a "gift" and have thought: Right. Show me to the exchange counter, and make it snappy. So I wince. Jennie catches my look and leans into the conversation.

"He talks!" she says, shaking her head and smiling. "Finally, finally, he tells me what he needs. You have no idea how wonderful this is." Jennie says she now has access to the father she never knew. She is able, she tells me, to be affectionate with him for the first time, to feel a part of his life, to feel necessary. She likes this changed man. Visiting him at Maplewood, she says, is "uplifting." I'm betting that not too many of the 10 million family members of Alzheimer's patients out there share Jennie's attitude. I'm betting that many would be shocked by the idea that she likes her father better with Alzheimer's than without. But I am not shocked. I am awed. There is a lesson here.

At work later that week, Eloise asks me if there are any vacant rooms in Maplewood, and when I say yes, she asks me whether I think Barbara would like to move in. Not a day goes by without her asking if I know Barbara, or if I will call Barbara, or if I know when Barbara will visit next. Barbara is one of Eloise's two daughters, the one who lives in town. I don't know when Barbara visits, but it's not when I'm on duty. In the month and a half I've been in the neighborhood, I haven't seen her. I've heard stories, though. She has a reputation among the RAs, and it's not a good one. They say Barbara is quick to find fault and stingy with kind words. She comes in, they say, with a chip on her shoulder, looking for problems: Eloise's bed is not made. Eloise isn't wearing lipstick. There was no caregiver in the neighborhood for ten minutes. The dinner was cold.

I have no doubt that Barbara sees what she says she sees. All these things happen, and more. We are overworked and understaffed—but never, I have to say emphatically, *never* intentionally negligent and never, ever cruel. I've seen the same elder-abuse stories on TV as everyone else, and I'm sure those filthy places staffed by nasty people actually exist. But this isn't one of them. I think Barbara may be unpopular with the RAs and administrative staff because they think she thinks we are one of these bad places. But if Eloise's dinner was cold on the day Barbara visited, it was because some stretched-way-too-thin RA was busy hand-feeding another resident. If Eloise's bed didn't get made, it was because the laundry had piled up, and the RA figured it was more important for residents to have clean clothes than for Eloise to have a neat bed. One caregiver in the neighborhood is not nearly enough. And so we find ourselves scrimping on the niceties to take care of the necessities. I think we need more people like Barbara, more family members who see faults in the eldercare system and make a fuss about it. But it's never pleasant to be on the receiving end of someone making the fuss.

Susan, the upbeat activity lady, does not allow herself to say anything bad about anybody, so when I ask about Barbara, she crimps her lips shut. Brooke, the imperturbable administrator, rolls her eyes. *Very challenging,* she says slowly, and walks away before she says anything more. I decide to give Barbara a call. She seems so much the antithesis of Jennie—the Witch of the West to Jennie's Glinda, the Good. I'd like to see myself as Glinda, but I fear I have more in common with the lady with the flying monkeys.

When I call Barbara at home to ask if we can meet for coffee, she is breathtakingly blunt. "Why should I spend my time talking to you?" she asks. I'm taken aback. People just don't talk that way. But I have to give her points for honesty. Most people want to be liked too much to be that honest. I make my pitch: I enjoy Eloise, I tell her. She is one of my favorites, and I'd like to know more about her. Barbara says she doesn't want to talk about her mother but reluctantly agrees to give me fifteen minutes one afternoon after my shift is over. I figure I've been interviewing people for twenty years. This woman is no match for me.

But, as it turns out, she is. Barbara is attractive in a Glenn Close kind of way, with cropped hair and a posture so erect I suspect spine-fusing surgery. I tell Barbara about my own mother, thinking to break the ice. But the ice is pretty thick. I tell her how much I like Eloise, how often Eloise speaks of her, but Barbara has her own agenda for our meeting. It appears that Barbara wants to persuade me to write an investigative article about Maplewood. She rails against the administrator, whom she says she can't stand. She criticizes the inadequate staffing and goes through a litany of lapses, oversights, and blunders she's seen during her visits. I wonder why Eloise is still at Maplewood if Barbara feels this way. When I ask her, she frowns. "They're all the same," she says. "All the facilities are the same."

I try, again and again, to steer the conversation toward Eloise. And I do manage to pick up a few biographical details, but the more I press, the more Barbara closes down. What I get from Barbara is anger. It is not directed at me, I know, but I feel its force. I also, all of a sudden, think I understand some of it. Yes, there are reasons to be angry at Maplewood—or at most any nursing home or assisted living center or Alzheimer's facility. The cost to families is high. The staff is generally undertrained and overworked. The turnover is astronomical, much like the profit realized by the big eldercare chains. But what Barbara is really angry at, I think, is her mother. How dare she get this disease. How dare she change from the globe-trotting, cruise-ship-sailing master bridge player that she was—I pick up at least these tidbits about her mother from Barbara—into a woman who wears diapers. How dare she need *me* as a mother when I'm not finished needing *her* as a mother. How dare she pass along a bad gene so that I might also become an old woman in diapers. The truth is, I can hear this loud and clear under Barbara's anger because I have felt the same way, because I said the same things to myself when it was my mother with the disease.

By the time my mother has been out West for two months, I am visiting her three or four times a week, down from the daily visits I had been making when she first arrived. It gets harder and harder. I can see that she's slipping. The biggest problem right now is her weight, her decreasing weight, which is ironic because during my childhood my mother was always either on a diet or planning a diet or beating herself up for cheating on a diet as she struggled to keep her weight at a number she invested with magical qualities: 120. At 120 pounds, everything was possible: straight skirts, slinky black dresses, bathing suits, the occasional admiring look from someone other than her husband.

She had been an ever-so-slightly-plump teenager—I've seen the pictures—who spent the rest of her life obsessed with her weight. Who knew better than her daughter the lifelong love-hate relationship she had with food? All those years, those decades, of dry toast and black coffee for breakfast, nonfat cottage cheese topped with chopped celery for lunch, Metrical and a side salad for dinner, no dessert, never any dessert. Cigarettes were her snack food. When I was a kid, I would sometimes catch her staring at herself in the full-length mirror on her closet door, sucking in her cheeks, pulling in her stomach, squinting and then scowling at what she saw.

And all the while she was cooking: fabulous dinners of beef bourguignon and coq au vin, pot roast in thick vegetable gravy, scampi, lamb chops with mint jelly, pork loin studded with garlic, scaloppini pounded paper thin and wrapped around prosciutto and Fontina, each little roll sewn together with thread. Even her meatloaf was wonderful. She cooked and she dieted, cooked and dieted, spending long afternoons creating meals she hardly let herself eat. Now, without trying, she was down to 110. She had, for the first time in her life, thin thighs.

Now she has to be fattened up. The caregivers at the facility are supplementing her meals with a high-calorie drink. If my mother knew she was downing a thick chocolate shake twice a day and still losing weight, she'd think she'd died and gone to heaven.

11

The third time this morning that Eloise asks about Barbara, I tell her a new lie. The old lie, that Barbara is at work and can't be reached right now, is not working. So I tell Eloise that I'm going to go out to the front desk and call Barbara. I walk out of the neighborhood and stand by the threshold of the door, just out of view. Then, as I count slowly to sixty, I think about what to do next.

"Okay," I tell Eloise when I come back in, "I just called Barbara." I watch her face change from tense to tranquil, like someone flipped a switch. She unhunches her bony shoulders. I hear her take a deep breath. "Barbara is out of town," I tell her. "But I talked to Tom."

"Oh yes, Tom," Eloise says. She remembers her son-in-law. This makes the call real for her.

"Tom says that Barbara is out of town at a conference," I tell Eloise, making it up as I go along. "She'll be gone for a few days, but she promises to come see you the moment she gets home." Eloise understands that her daughter works, that she has a career. She knows about out-of-town conferences. She is satisfied with this explanation.

"You are so good to me," she says. I wonder.

But I don't have much time to ponder personal ethics this morning. Anxiety is in the air. I think sometimes that mood is contagious, that residents spread nervousness and unease among each other like sniffles. Whatever the etiology, Eloise is not the only one who's jittery today. Marianne, generally calm and composed, needs my attention. She is pacing the neighborhood, dressed in her usual professional woman clothes, carrying her handbag.

"Have you seen Frank?" she asks me. I don't remember who Frank is to Marianne, but that doesn't matter right now.

"No, I'm afraid I haven't seen him," I say. "But you know, I don't get out of this section of the building very much, Marianne." *Section of the building.* That's part of the code I use when I talk to Marianne. It allows us to talk about this place without using words that identify it for what it really is.

"Well," Marianne says, "I don't know what his schedule is, but I assume we're dining together." I nod pleasantly. "When he arrives, please direct him to my office." Ten minutes later, she finds me folding laundry in the living area. "Have you seen Frank?" she asks. I say no. "I'll just check downstairs to see if he's arrived yet," she tells me. There is no downstairs here. Marianne is always so confident in her delusions, so articulate, so precise, that it sometimes makes me doubt my own version of reality. Maybe there *is* a downstairs here. Maybe her room *is* her office. Maybe she *does* work here. Maybe Frank, whoever he is, *is* waiting to take her to lunch.

The noon meal has arrived by cart, and I start lifting the domed covers from the plastic dinner plates. Underneath, the food is, mysteriously, always room temperature, regardless of what it is and when it left the kitchen. As I distribute the plates, I try to persuade Marianne that she should sit down at the table with everyone else. Perhaps Frank meant that you were to meet *after* lunch, I suggest. Perhaps he wants to get together for coffee. She considers this.

"That may be so," she says. Her voice trails off. I can't help getting the feeling that Marianne is losing faith in this Frank scenario. If so, this calls my role into question. If Marianne, in a moment of clarity, has realized that Frank isn't coming to pick her up, if she has suddenly remembered that Frank in fact died a while ago (I checked Marianne's file before lunch: Frank was her husband, and he has been dead since the late '90s), then she might look at me and wonder: Who is this woman pretending that Frank may show up after lunch? *I* become the crazy one.

Marianne eats quickly. She has so much to do, she tells me. She has to get home and take care of things, she says. She wants to leave me a note with names on it, her "contacts." I find her a piece of paper. She walks off with it, returning a few minutes later to ask if Frank has called, if he's left a message. She's agitated, but not in that needy way Eloise is when she's agitated. Marianne is more like a harried executive with too much on her plate and too little confidence in her subordinates, of which, I believe, she considers me one. I tell her there is no phone in here, but I will check at the main desk to see if any messages came in. It's exhausting playing along with these scenarios. Some days I lie so much that I forget my own lies.

The next day, Marianne is agitated again. The first thing she says when she sees me is that she is expecting a phone call. "I don't know from whom, and I don't know when," she says, which, I can see by the way she raises her eyebrows, sounds strange even to her. She wants to make sure the call comes through. She wants me to alert the front desk. I tell her that I will, which of course, I won't. A few minutes later, she tells me, as she did yesterday, that she has so many things to accomplish that she will need to go home.

"Do you need me around here tomorrow, or have you got things under control?" she asks. I tell her that whatever she needs to do tomorrow is just fine with me. "So my plans will work with your schedule?" she asks, making sure. It's clear to me how she is experiencing this moment: she is an administrator who will be away from the office for a day, and she's checking with an underling (me) to make sure the office will run smoothly in her absence. I guess we're back to the delusion in which Maplewood is some sort of workplace and not the delusion in which Maplewood is a corporate retreat for female execs. I wonder if there are other ways Marianne experiences this place and how I will keep up with all of them. I assure her again that I have tomorrow covered. Sometimes I am concerned that feeding her delusions may ultimately be harmful; other times I feel certain that for Marianne, living in a fantasy world is a protection, a solace, and I cannot destroy that.

Inez, the Med Aide on duty today, comes around with everyone's pills: vitamins, diuretics, blood thinners, stool softeners, beta-blockers, pills for high blood pressure, low blood pressure, diabetes, osteoporosis. It's the rare resident who is not on some kind of medication. A number of people here take Aricept, one of the FDA-approved drugs for Alzheimer's. When these medications are effective at all—my mother took Cognex, another of these drugs, and it helped not a whit—they may slow mental decline by a few months. None of them can stop, or reverse, the progression of the disease. All of them work to mitigate symptoms, not attack the cause.

There are new drugs out there in the FDA pipeline, medications that may help prevent the buildup of plaque or reduce inflammation or boost the levels of neurotransmitters—that is, attack the causes of Alzheimer's. There are drugs being tested that harness the immune system to attack brain-clogging plaque, or that activate the "janitor" cells that normally mop up excess gluey protein, or that use the brain's own chemistry to block the production of toxins now thought to be part of the chain of events leading to Alzheimer's. There's an experimental drug that might actually help create long-term memory. There's intriguing new evidence that marijuana (TCH, that is) and red wine might inhibit the progress of the disease. There's the hint that statins might work, the promise of a memory vaccine, the dream of gene therapy. But right now, for the folks who live at Maplewood and for the millions of others who have Alzheimer's, there are just a few stop-gap medications.

I ask Inez and another Med Aide if they think those taking the Alzheimer's medications are doing any better than those who aren't. They say they can't tell the difference. That's not to say the drugs don't work for some people. I'm sure they do. The clinical trials show they do. But the difference the drug makes—when it makes a difference—the slowing in the rate of decline, can be pretty subtle. It's also true that each person declines at his or her own rate. Eloise, who is not taking an Alzheimer's drug, seems the same to me now as she did more than a year ago when I first started observing here. My mother, on the other hand, took a memory drug and declined so rapidly that within five months it was hard to believe she was the same person. Also, the individual rate of decline, whatever it is, may be neither steady nor predictable. A person can reach a plateau, stay there for a long while, and then decline precipitously. For people with Alzheimer's living at home—not in a clinical setting, where patients are given standardized tests at frequent intervals—it is very hard to judge something like rate of decline. Still, families want to feel they are doing *something*. My mother kept taking Cognex long after we realized it wasn't doing anything, or anything discernible. It was the *idea* of the drug, not the reality. If she stopped the drug, it meant we were giving up hope.

Marianne is taking heart-disease medication and, as of today, Aricept. She balks when Inez hands her the pills. "I don't take anything unless I know exactly what it is," she tells Inez, which seems perfectly reasonable to me. Inez doesn't get it. Inez is used to dealing with people who are much farther gone than Marianne.

"Look," she says, holding out the pill. "It's just a tiny one. Very easy to take."

"That is not the point," says Marianne. "I will only take what is prescribed by my own physician." Now Inez gets it.

"This *is* prescribed by your doctor."

"Then you can please tell me exactly what I am taking," Marianne says. Her voice is calm, but she is clearly annoyed, clearly aware that she is not being treated like the perfectly competent professional she believes herself to be. Then, before Inez answers, Marianne turns to Sandy, the Float who has come into the neighborhood to give me my ten-minute break. "I am being overmedicated, and this has to stop," she says. This just isn't true. Marianne takes only two pills a day for her heart condition. She does not take antidepressants or antipsychotics or any kind of mood-altering meds. This is, in fact, a point of real, and justified, pride at Maplewood. We work hard to control behaviors—anxiety, anger, restlessness—without pharmaceuticals. We substitute music, activities, touch, and warm cookies for Xanax, Valium and Ativan. If people walk around Maplewood in a trance, it's Alzheimer's induced, not drug induced. And so I think Marianne's concern may just be paranoia. I know that paranoia sometimes accompanies Alzheimer's. Or maybe Marianne remembers herself as a healthy person who doesn't take any medication, so that two pills seem like a lot.

Sandy starts to explain the Aricept to her, telling her that it's a memory drug, that it helps slow memory loss. I am looking hard at Marianne, trying to determine how she's taking this information. As far as I've been able to discern, she isn't aware that she has memory loss. Certainly she has no idea she has been diagnosed with Alzheimer's or that she is living in an Alzheimer's care facility. She is listening hard.

"My doctor came up with this pill?" Marianne asks, interrupting Sandy.

I would have just answered yes, been done with the conversation, and handed her the damned pill. But Sandy plays it differently. She explains that other doctors elsewhere did the research and developed the medication. Marianne nods. She considers this information, but she is clearly baffled. "How did these doctors know about *me*?" she asks Sandy. I suppress a smile and move in closer to see what Sandy does with this question. Sandy doesn't see the whimsy. She makes a halting attempt at explaining research protocols. Marianne has lost interest.

"But my doctor knows about this pill and wants me to take it?" she asks, interrupting Sandy again. Assured that this is so, she swallows it, then turns to me. "I'm expecting a very important phone call this afternoon," she says. "I'll be in my office. Please make sure I am notified when it comes through."

These days I think more and more about alternative realities, about the different worlds inhabited by the people I care for. I have long understood that reality is subjective, that, for example, the mother-child conversation I experience as well-meaning and inspirational can be to my teenage son invasive and embarrassing. But at least we both agree we were in the car together that afternoon, that it was raining hard, that a Green Day CD was playing, that we were mother and son on an errand. We experienced the moment differently, but not *so* differently, not Marianne-differently.

When I allow myself to accept these other realities—Marianne's I'm-an-administrator-here vision of her life, Hayes's precise, narrow, mechanistic world—or when I myself create other realities—the ongoing fiction of phoning Eloise's daughter Barbara—I begin to experience a paradigm shift. It is a shift away from disease, disability, and dementia, and toward "personhood," a concept I read about in a groundbreaking British book called *Dementia Reconsidered*. Tom Kitwood, the geriatric psychologist who wrote the book in the late 1990s, believes simply, and powerfully, that "the person comes first," that attention to personhood rather than pathology could, and should, revolutionize Alzheimer's care. In fact, the book has had a major impact on Alzheimer's care in Great Britain but not, it seems, in the United States. I think *Dementia Reconsidered* is quietly brilliant and as radical a treatise on disease as Susan Sontag's far more famous—and far less readable—work. Kitwood's idea helps me look at Marianne or Eloise or Hayes or any of the others as interesting people, not as—or at least not *only* as—victims of an illness. It's not that I forget they have Alzheimer's. It's that, with the paradigm shifted, the disease no longer defines them. They are who they are *and* they have Alzheimer's.

This doesn't seem like a lesson I—or anyone else—would still need to learn. The disability-rights folks have been telling us this for decades: I am a person with a disability. I am not a disability. I am not Jane Jones, the paraplegic. I am Jane Jones, and my legs are paralyzed. It's not a matter of politically correct speech. It's not semantics. It is actually a different way of looking at people.

The next morning, delusional, cantankerous Frances M. is in a helping mood, which means I have to keep my eye on her all the time. When I disappear for a moment to take Pam into her room to use the commode, I return to find Frances M. wheeling Addie away from the breakfast table, only Addie is not ready to go. Her plate is full of food. She is grasping a triangle of toast in her hand. I smile, pat Frances M. on the back, and thank her extravagantly—maintaining her good mood is a priority—and wheel Addie back to the table. I get a few bites of scrambled egg into her. While she chews, I walk Frances M. to her place at the table, pull back her chair with an exaggerated flourish, and make encouraging remarks about eating breakfast. Then I go back to feeding Addie.

Seconds later, I see that Frances M. is up again and has now started to wheel Hayes away from his table. I stop what I'm doing and go over there. I tell Frances that Hayes needs to eat. I put a piece of toast in his hand.

"What do I do now?" he asks.

"You eat the toast," I say, forgetting that Hayes needs more specific directions. He is motionless. Frances hovers, shifting her weight from foot to foot. I try again. "You take the toast and put it in your mouth, and you chew it," I say. Then I take hold of the hand with the toast and guide it to his mouth. He doesn't open his lips. I instruct him to open his mouth, then I push a corner of toast past his teeth. "Now chew," I say. He chews. I go back to Addie.

When I look over my shoulder maybe a minute later, Frances M. is helping Hayes eat. She is feeding him his hot cereal with a fork. The cream of wheat is dribbling between the tines onto his clean blue sweater and making its way in sluggish white rivulets down his front to his khakis. My first thought is just how long it's going to take to get Hayes back to his room, out of his wheelchair, into fresh clothes, back into his wheelchair, and out to the common area. I am about to rush over to shoo Frances away—I mean *redirect her*, as we say in the biz—when I realize something else is going on: Frances M. and Hayes are sitting together companionably and talking. The conversation goes like this:

Hayes: Help me. Are you helping me?

Frances M.: Oh yes. This is right. I'm ready now.

Hayes: My back is itchy. It is so itchy.

Frances M.: Deanne will be late for school. I have to do something.

Hayes: I'm Hayes. Hayes Bottoms. Everyone has a bottom.

It sounds crazy. It makes no sense if you pay attention to the words. But if you listen instead to the tone and the voice patterns, if you look at the body language, then it seems very much like a conversation. He asks. She answers. He comments. She comments. They take turns. They look at each other. Clearly they are connecting. I think about the notion of "excessive talkativity," another phrase coined by the British Alzheimer's guru Tom Kitwood. We are so focused on words, he says, on the act of talking, that we have forgotten how to communicate without them. More than that, we think there is no communication without words—which, of course, means that we believe we can't communicate with those who, in the later throes of Alzheimer's, have lost most of their language. These sentences Hayes and Frances M. say to each other may not make sense as conversation, yet there is meaning here. Frances stops fidgeting for a moment. Hayes stops calling for help. They are getting something out of this moment. They are partners in an alternate reality.

I go over and give Frances M. a hug. She is not ordinarily very huggable. "You're having such a good day today," I tell her.

"I'm a human being today," she says.

12

Eloise is having a hard time yet again this morning. Barbara is the daughter she obsesses about most days, but Eloise also has a younger daughter who lives in Chicago, where Eloise used to live before she came here, where Eloise owned a lovely house and had a kind husband and lived a good life playing bridge and going on cruises. Earlier this morning, Eloise's Chicago daughter called. She calls with the best of intentions, out of love and filial devotion, out of a need to stay in touch and stay connected. But what happens is these phone calls remind Eloise that she used to have another life. They jolt her out of the seamless present, the days spent in the neighborhood listening to music or napping under a quilt or having her nails done or sitting at the dining room table drinking decaf. Her daughter calls and all of a sudden, Eloise remembers Chicago and that this place in which she now lives is not her home.

Eloise is sitting in her room, perched on the edge of her bed. "I want to go home," she says. This is her bitter-combative voice, not her usual pleasant I-am-a-lady voice.

"You *are* home," I tell her, putting a hand on her knee. "*This* is your home."

"No. It. Is. Not." says Eloise. She enunciates each word, as if talking to someone stupid or slow.

I try to reason with her. "Eloise, look around at your room. These are all your things. This has been your home for almost a year now." I can read the frustration in her face. She *knows* she is not home. She is thinking about her house, where she raised her daughters. She is thinking about Chicago. She narrows her eyes and shoots me a dirty look.

"I just want to go HOME!" she yells.

I hate to see Eloise so upset. It makes me feel sad and helpless. Sometimes I think Addie, or even Rose, is better off than Eloise because for them there's no tension between what used to be and what is. What used to be is inaccessible, invisible through the thick fog of Alzheimer's. What used to be is gone. But Eloise can sometimes see through the fog, like today. Maybe I can distract her, redirect her, get her thinking about something else. "How about a cup of tea?" I ask her. "I bet I can find one of those sugar cookies I baked yesterday."

Eloise stares at me as if I am the enemy. "No. I want to go home."

"Maybe you'd like to take a little nap?"

"Don't talk to me about anything else!" Eloise yells. "I want to go home!"

Clearly I am doing harm here, not good. Eloise is more agitated now than she was when I walked in the room. Best to leave her alone for a few minutes. I've got chores to do, people to check on. Maybe she will work herself out of this mood. Maybe the fog will roll in.

A few minutes later I see Eloise walk out of her room and head for the kitchen area where a teenage volunteer is wiping the counter. Occasionally we'll get someone from the nearby high school who wants to earn community service hours. It's wonderful to have another set of hands around the neighborhood, if only for an hour or two. The girls—all the volunteers are girls—do everything from helping to serve meals to giving amateur manicures to running for supplies. Eloise looks at the young woman.

"Can you do something for me?" she asks. It's the sweet voice.

"Sure," says the volunteer. "What is it?"

"Get me out of here. I want to go home." Eloise spits out each word. The high school girl looks over at me for help, but I don't know what to do either. I know I've got to come up with some new approach, not only for Eloise's sake but for the neighborhood's. This is one of those moods that can be contagious.

Dottie, whose room is on one side of Eloise's, hears the commotion and comes out to the kitchen. Dottie is the former volleyball champ who plays a mean game of balloon ball, the one with the overhand serve that propels the ball almost out of the neighborhood. She will be eighty-eight next month, but with her compact, meat-on-the-bones body and her creamy skin, she could pass for sixty-five. Dottie happily participates in all the group activities but otherwise keeps her own counsel. She is so self-contained and self-reliant that some days I hardly know she's here. I have, in fact, wondered *why* she's here. She seems competent. Her language is good. She doesn't appear confused. Unlike Marianne, who is also competent and articulate, Dottie seems to know exactly where she is and why. She does have memory problems, but as far as I can tell, they are the kind of problems anyone her age might have: She can't recall the birth date of a grandchild. She's not quite sure what years she lived in which towns.

Dottie has apparently been listening and watching as this

scene with Eloise is playing out. She assesses the situation and takes over. Eloise has now decided that she must call her Chicago daughter. She will simply tell her daughter that she wants to go home. Her daughter will come and pick her up, and that will be that. I know better than to try to explain to Eloise why this is not going to happen, that things simply do not work this way. I think Dottie knows that Eloise's plan is not possible, but she goes along with Eloise's fiction. Or maybe Dottie doesn't know. She must live at Maplewood for *some* reason.

Dottie corrals Eloise, and the two of them walk back to Eloise's room to make the phone call. Eloise is the only person in the neighborhood to have a private phone. There are jacks in all the rooms, and the option is open to anyone, but family members don't often pay for phone service. It's not an amenity most residents need—or would even be aware of. Eloise's phone is there, I think, for the express purpose of receiving calls from her Chicago daughter.

Dottie and Eloise sit on her bed with the phone between them. Eloise is holding the receiver. Dottie is punching the numbers. They sit like this for a minute, two minutes, three minutes. I lean against the door frame and watch them. They are talking in low tones, conspiring. Dottie is laughing about how she can't figure out how to use the phone. Is Dottie pretending? If so, it's a wonderful, generous pretense. The act of trying to make the phone call empowers Eloise. She is doing something. She has control. She is not just listening to people tell her what she doesn't want to hear. And this begins to calm her. It doesn't seem to matter that the call is not going through, that Dottie is just pressing random buttons. Eloise is involved in this moment with her friend. She is sitting on her bed having a little talk with Dottie. Her anxiety ebbs.

A few minutes later, Eloise and Dottie emerge from the room.

Dottie pulls up two chairs, and they sit side by side at the kitchen counter. I serve them cups of Lipton tea. Dottie pats Eloise's hand. I think that maybe Eloise has forgotten everything already.

But when Eloise looks over at Dottie, I see I am wrong. Eloise is calm now, but she looks embarrassed. She knows she has carried on. She knows she's made a fuss. And the part of her that is refined and well-bred, the part of her that is still very much the Eloise she used to be, is appalled. "I am *so* sorry," Eloise says to Dottie. "Something just comes over me." Dottie nods. Then she reaches over to pat her friend's hand again.

Soon after I clock in for my shift the next morning, I get a call on the walkie from Patty, the receptionist, telling me to check 129's bathroom. That's the one Frances M. and Jane share. Jane is the little fireplug of a woman who is at the center of social activity in the neighborhood, the one whose keys I found in the dryer. There's a pull cord in each bathroom that residents can use if they get into trouble. When the cord is pulled it activates an alert system in the reception area, and a light goes on under a room number. Apparently, the light is on under 129. I am in Eloise's room when I get the call. I leave her sitting on her bed half-dressed and rush across the common area.

There, in the bathroom, sits Jane on the floor, her back against the tile wall, her legs bent to the side. I see Jane, but all I can think of is Ella. *This is going to be another Ella. Jane is going to die just like Ella.* I barely knew Ella—I had just started working here when she fell that morning—but I know Jane. She's the little engine that could, tough and feisty, a joker, a talker. She doesn't have Eloise's sweetness, but then again she doesn't have Eloise's moods. In fact, she has only one mood: good.

Among Jane's roles in the neighborhood are Greeter of New Residents, Listener of Life Stories, and Keeper of the Birds. It is

Jane I count on to come to the table and make conversation with the new arrival, the woman who now lives in Ella's old room. It is Jane who listens to Pam, lets her talk on and on as her stories get more tangled and less sensible. And it is Jane who, every morning, awakens the birds, the three parakeets who live in an oversized cage set against the living room wall. She removes and folds the sheet that has been draped over the cage for the night, clicking her tongue at the birds, rousing them with an encouraging little chirp.

Jane has a litany of health problems—congestive heart failure, hypertension, anemia—but you wouldn't know it. Built square, solid, and close to the ground, she has a happy, alert face, good color, a hearty appetite, and an intact sense of humor. One morning we ran out of Rice Krispies, her breakfast mainstay, and I served her cornflakes instead. She pretended to be upset, pushed the bowl away, and told me she was going to fire me. A few minutes later she stuffed a Tootsie Roll in the pocket of my half-apron. Another morning I was late with the breakfasts because after Hayes was already out at the table and seated, he announced he had to go to the bathroom. Even when everything goes right with this venture, it takes almost ten minutes. And rarely does everything go right. When I returned, wheeling Hayes in front of me, Jane followed me into the kitchen, chucked me on the arm, and shook her head in mock disapproval. "So while our breakfasts are getting cold you're out gallivanting with this handsome guy," she said.

And now Jane is on the bathroom floor. It turns out that she slipped on a wet spot caused by Frances M., who apparently wandered into the bathroom sometime during the night and turned on the shower. She didn't turn it on full force, otherwise the noc-shift RA surely would have noticed. The water is just trickling from the showerhead, but because there is no lip or ledge between the shower and the floor—that's so people in wheelchairs or using walkers can get in and out easily—the trickle has spread out across the floor.

Jane looks up at me and smiles. She doesn't seem too upset. She just can't maneuver herself to get up, she tells me, otherwise she never would have pulled the cord. She's talking and smiling, and I'm thinking: *broken hip, hospital, she'll never get out alive.* I call for help and kneel down to talk to her. I don't want to move her in case she has, in fact, broken something. Meanwhile, Frances M., who was downright nasty yesterday, hovers solicitously in the doorway. Jane tells me that Frances tried to help. That would have been interesting to watch.

Jasmine, who is working the neighborhood next door today and has followed the interchange on her walkie-talkie, comes in to help. A minute later, the Med Aide on duty arrives. She takes Jane's vitals, which are fine, and inspects her arms, legs, and torso for cuts or bruises, of which there are none (yet). Jane is impatient. She moves both arms in big circles, extends her legs and then pulls them back, bending her knees. "See," she says, "just fine." Jane is proud of her independence. She hates that she's fallen but not as much as she hates that we're making a big deal about it. The Med Aide feels a goose egg on the back of Jane's head. Jane reluctantly admits that her back hurts a little.

We ease her upright. This will tell the tale. If she can't support her weight, then something could very well be broken. Jasmine holds one arm; I grab the other. Jane wobbles for a moment, finds her balance, and takes a step. I don't realize that I've been holding my breath until I hear myself exhale. Jane takes another step and another, then she shrugs off our support. We bookend her as she moves toward the door to her room, close enough to touch but not touching. Jasmine gives me a thumbs-up. The Med Aide returns with two extra-strength Tylenol. She's already called Jane's doctor to schedule an X-ray.

Jane stays in her room all morning. She has her own TV in there and a comfortable armchair by the window. I check on her several times. The Med Aide checks on her. Jasmine comes over on her ten-minute break and sits with her for a few minutes. It seems everything is going to be okay. But when Jane comes out for lunch, she is walking very slowly and wincing a little with each step. I call the Med Aide on the walkie. She tells me that Jane will go out for her X-ray after lunch.

Pam has been watching Jane's slow progress across the room. Pam is a worrier. I think she's probably always been a worrier. With seven kids to raise, the last four as a single mother, she probably worried for good reason. In here she doesn't have much to worry about beyond making sure her walker doesn't get tangled in the tubing that goes from her oxygen tank to the little contraption under her nose. But she nevertheless manages to find something to worry about every day. Today she doesn't have to look hard.

As soon as Jane settles in, Pam comes over, pushing her walker, and pulls up a chair next to her. "I'm going to take care of you," she tells Jane, and hunches in close. Then Marianne, who was sitting at the far end of the table, gets up, walks over, and pulls up a chair on the other side. This is surprising. If the neighborhood had a Warm Woman competition, Marianne might come in last. She is so concerned with herself, her room, the appointments she thinks she has, the phone calls she thinks she's expecting, that she rarely interacts with the others. Or maybe it's just that she's keeping a proper distance between herself—the administrator—and everyone else (underlings) here. Whatever the case, Marianne does not extend herself. It's a testament to

Jane's place in the neighborhood, her centrality to the social scene, that Marianne is by her side. She takes Jane's hand and pats it. Pam, not to be outdone, grabs Jane's forearm and strokes it.

And there they sit, the three of them, shoulder to shoulder, two friends consoling a third. I stand back and watch, not wanting to intrude into this moment. I catch myself thinking, *Why, it's just like real life.* Then I realize, it *is* real life.

But it is soon obvious that Marianne has depleted her small store of goodwill on the exchange with Jane. After spending the first half of lunch quietly and kindly commiserating with her friend, she turns the full force of her attention to Hayes. Hayes is being his usual demanding self, calling out *Help me, won't somebody help me* every fifteen seconds, even when I am right there in the act of helping him. He is, as usual, driving everyone nuts. Marianne gets out of her seat next to Jane at the main table and carries her plate over to the four-person table where Hayes always sits. At first just her presence quiets him. Or maybe he's just too surprised to speak. I come over at regular intervals to feed him in between tending to Addie and Old Frances. His silence doesn't last long.

"I need help here," he calls out seconds after I leave him to help Addie. As I feed her—which first involves waking her up as she falls asleep between bites—I hear Marianne start to lecture Hayes. She adopts a superior, scolding voice, like an old-fashioned fussy lady teacher talking to an errant fourth grader. She tells him he's rude, that he needs to be considerate of others. I listen carefully for his response, wondering what he'll say, wondering what is registering.

He looks at Marianne, his eyes vacant and innocent. "I can't hear anything you're saying," he says pleasantly. Marianne takes that as an invitation to repeat herself, only louder, and launches into a reprise of her civility lecture. Hayes is looking down at his lap chewing a bite of hamburger, crumbles of which are edging out the corner of his mouth and getting stuck between his neck and the collar of his plaid shirt. Marianne senses that she's not making any headway and decides to change her approach.

"You know," she says affably, or as affably as Marianne gets, "I think you are really deep down a kind man."

Hayes stops chewing. "Kind man," he says, nodding. Now, all of a sudden, he hears just fine.

"But today you are very rude, very rude," she says. I go over, hand Hayes his glass of milk, position the straw between his lips, and then rush back to feeding Addie before she falls asleep again. I can hear Marianne still at it, telling Hayes that he's not the only person in the dining room, that we are all tired of listening to him, that he ought to control himself. All of which is true. But Hayes is Hayes. He is pared down to the essential Hayes, and nothing Marianne says, nothing I do, will change that. She's going on and on, but talking in a softer voice now, a normal conversational tone.

I figure Hayes can't hear her or has tuned her out. But when I come over again to feed him another bite, he looks up at me with his big, watery eyes and says, sweetly, "I don't think that lady likes me very much."

13

Hayes does not want to get up this morning. And when Hayes doesn't want to do something, he is a force to be reckoned with. I've found that it's better to wait him out. I wish I could put a CD in his machine, let him snooze in bed, get him up later, and serve him a reheated breakfast. It would make my life much easier. But that's not an option this morning because Hayes has managed to soak his bed. His pajamas are wet, even, somehow, the tops. The absorbent pad we put between him and his flannel sheets is wet, as are the sheets, both top and bottom. Even his blanket is damp to the touch. The only dry thing about Hayes is, miraculously, his Depends. They hang rakishly from his right hip, the adhesive tab on the other side long since detached. I wonder if the noc-shift caregiver did her last check before she clocked out—or any check, for that matter. This looks like a full night's worth of peeing to me.

I can't leave Hayes resting between cold, wet sheets, regardless of how much of a fuss he's making. I've got to get him up and out of bed. He'll need a shower before I can dress him in clean, dry clothes. I rush to the bathroom to start the shower, find towels in his cabinet, and set them out. Hayes wants to know what I'm doing, what's going on. Whatever it is, he doesn't like it. He resists my efforts to lift him into a sitting position in bed, but I finally get him upright. I should have brought his walker over to the bed before I did this, but I forgot. Now, looking around his room as I support him with one arm, I can't see the walker anywhere. It must be out in the common area. I prop him up on his two (damp) pillows and tell him I'll be right back. He is not pleased.

"I'm cold," he says testily. "I'm so cold." I find a lap blanket near his chair and wrap it around his shoulders. "Where are you going?" he yells after me. I tell him. "Will I see you later?" Sometimes this guy is just impossible.

Yes, I say, with a big sigh, in just a minute.

"See you later, agitator," he calls after me, singsong. How does he do that? How does he know just when to get all charming?

I rush back in with his walker and begin the elaborate multistep process—with the accompanying play-by-play commentary that Hayes demands—of standing him up, walking him to the bathroom, taking off his clothes, sitting him on the plastic stool in his shower, washing him, et cetera, et cetera.

"What are we doing now?" Hayes asks the one time out of ten that I've neglected to give him the blow-by-blow. He's finally clean and toweled dry. I am carefully positioning his arm in the sleeve of a fresh undershirt. It's barely 7:00 a.m. and I'm exhausted already. I wish he would cut me some slack.

"I'm changing you," I tell him. I don't even try to mask my exasperation.

"Changing me into what?" asks Hayes.

_____

Hayes is at his best when Mabel, his wife of sixty-eight years, visits. One of their children, usually Jennie, drives Mabel out to Maplewood two or three times a week. Sometimes Mabel sits with him during the mid-morning events Susan organizes, like "Sing-Along with Helen" or "Piano with Trudy" or "Accordion Plus with Bernie." Susan is a music lover. The Maplewood calendar is jammed with interactive sings and instrumental performances, a parade of good-hearted elderly musicians of varying talents who make the rounds from Alzheimer's centers to assisted living facilities to nursing homes. It's a circuit, like the Catskills.

Hayes taps his bony fingers on his bony thigh in time to the music. Mabel sits close with a faint, dazed smile on her lips. She is almost ninety, a year and a half younger than Hayes, and, although she seems to be in good health both mentally and physically, she hasn't quite grasped—or maybe admitted to herself—that something is wrong with her husband.

Today, after enjoying a morning concert billed as "Julie at her Organ," Mabel stays for lunch. I love it on the days she stays for lunch. Sometimes she feeds Hayes or encourages him to feed himself. But even when she just sits next to him at the little table silently eating her own plate of lukewarm Maplewood mystery meat, she is a godsend. Hayes is quiet during those meals. There are no every-ten-second outbursts of *help me, won't somebody help me* or *I'm itchy, I'm itchy.* I can tend to the others. Everyone eats in peace.

After lunch I wheel Hayes into his bathroom to take care of business. Mabel walks around his room, plumping pillows, touching knickknacks, not knowing what to do with herself. When I get him back into his big blue chair by the window, she tucks a blanket around his legs, sits on the chair next to him, and reaches for his hand. Their marriage has been a long and faithful one. This is a woman who loves her husband. Hayes looks at her for a long moment. He is clearly mystified. "Who *are* you?" he asks. The look that crosses her face is heartbreaking.

When I peek in a few minutes later, Mabel is standing in front of Hayes's chair, holding both his hands in hers. Their arms are outstretched. She is swaying back and forth. His head cocks first to the left, then the right, then back again. Count Basie is playing on the CD. He is seated, but they are dancing.

I only pretended to feel love like this for my mother. In the first few years of her disease, when my father was caring for her by himself at home, I used to write long and what I thought of as heartfelt letters to him. I'd ask about the details of their life together, commiserate with him over the latest problem— bedwetting, wandering, weird behavior at the hair salon—and praise him for learning how to do all the domestic chores that had been done for him during forty-five years of marriage. One time my father showed one of my letters to a new neighbor, a middle-aged widow who I believe had designs on him. "I can't believe this is from your daughter," she said, or so he told me. "It's all head and no heart. Doesn't she care?"

She had a point, this neighbor-lady I'd never met who knew nothing about my mother and me. She was wrong about me not caring, but she was on to something. I *did* care—but from an emotional distance. I cared but not from that visceral place where love is.

When was I growing up, I admired my mother. She was prettier and smarter than all the other kids' mothers. She was different, too—worldlier. She played the piano; she painted still lifes in oil on canvasses she stretched herself in the basement, hammering together her own frames at the hobby bench my father never used. She designed an entire wardrobe for my favorite doll, hand sewing lines of snaps on all the enclosures, embroidering designs on the yokes of the dresses, finishing the inside seams. She designed and sewed all of my clothes, from Madras bermudas for summer camp to a spaghetti-strap crimson brocade for the junior prom. She designed the costumes for school plays. She refinished furniture, wove baskets, tiled counters, rewired lamps. She was a Block Mother and a Girl Scout leader. She recorded books for the blind.

She had energy and wit and style: the silk kerchief tied at the throat, the high heels she wore even to go food shopping, the straight skirts with kick pleats, the single eyebrow raised, a trick she perfected as a teenager after long hours in front of the mirror. She had beautiful eyebrows, high and arched, never plucked too thin. She had beautiful eyes, too, a clear, pale blue, with dark lashes that needed no mascara. When she raised a single eyebrow, she looked theatrical, sophisticated, European—and she knew it.

My mother was part of that Depression Era–World War II generation of women, twenty years too young to take strength from Alice Paul, twenty years too old to model themselves after Gloria Steinem. It was the generation of women who were told, when it suited the country, that they could do anything: drive a truck, run factory equipment, bring in the harvest.

My mother, who had a degree from Pratt in clothes design, was hired as a draftswoman to design the wings of warplanes. Every morning before she left her apartment, she used her sharp eye and her even hand to draw stocking seams on the backs of her bare legs. Eyebrow pencil worked best. All the women did it when they could no longer buy nylon stockings in the store. Nylon was needed for parachutes, for the boys. My mother had her own set of precision tools she brought to work in a small black leather case. She sat on a high stool in front of a big, slanted wooden table and did important work every day. She was good at it. She got bigger assignments. She was promoted several times until she became head of a twenty-person department. Then, in the fall of 1945, she was fired. The war was over. The men had come home. *Thanks, gals, now get back where you belong.*

My mother listened. She quickly married a returning GI and settled in for the long haul. By the time Betty Friedan's *Feminine Mystique* hit the bookstores, my mother was serving her second term as president of the local PTA and serving her family four-course home-cooked meals every night. She had two children, a tract house in the suburbs, a husband who doled out allowance to her every other Thursday night, and what I now know, in retrospect, was the beginning of a drinking problem.

During the war years, she had been an independent woman. When she wasn't designing airplane parts, she was flirting with French soldiers at a West Side Manhattan hangout called Pierre au Tunnel. She spoke beautiful French. She learned to drink Pernod. She had dreams starring herself and tall, dark, handsome men whose faces she couldn't quite make out.

By the mid-1960s, her hangout was the A&P on Wantagh Avenue, and her spirit was dampened by a decade of suburban isolation. She cooked, she sewed, she changed the bed linen every Monday, clipped coupons and went grocery shopping every Wednesday, ironed on Thursday, waxed the kitchen floor on Friday, and polished the wedding silver once a month.

For a while, a long while, she made efforts to hold on to who she was. Those were her most active days, my growing-up years, when she was Miracle Mother: gourmet cook, professional seamstress, interior decorator, parent leader, community volunteer. She taught an adult education class in dressmaking. She finished the *New York Times* crossword puzzle every day.

But no matter what she did, it didn't seem to be enough to sustain her. Her restlessness showed in her short temper and her long silences, in the way she seemed to grow colder, more detached, less focused every year. I don't know what her dreams were during those years, and I am not sure she knew either, at least not in the way women of later generations have known that they wanted to be veterinarians or cops, wanted to live in San Francisco or train for the Olympics. She just wanted excitement, I think, and romance. She wanted to be Bette Davis. She wanted Paul Henreid to put two cigarettes between his lips, light them both, and pass one to her.

Instead, she found herself behind the wheel of a two-tone DeSoto waiting to pick up her husband at the Long Island Rail Road station, living in a split-level, standing in line for her "house money" twice a month. And so, slowly, over the years, I think she began to forget who she was. She stopped painting. She stopped playing the piano. The dressmaker's dummy went down to the basement, and the sewing machine languished under an increasingly thick layer of dust. She stopped doing projects. She stopped volunteering. Instead, she sat in the club chair by the picture window reading Sidney Sheldon novels, chain-smoking Tareytons, and drinking vodka straight, no ice.

It seemed to me, watching this from afar, from college and beyond, that she was living a life she chose by acquiescence rather than decision. She stayed because that's what women of her generation did, because she didn't know she had other choices, because she was selfless, because she was scared, because she was lazy. She stayed out of love. She stayed out of a failure of imagination. The truth is, I don't know why she stayed. Me, I left. I moved across the continent and never looked back.

I don't know if there was a link between the life she led and the disease that shortened it. But there is one thing I am sure of:

she began to lose her self long before Alzheimer's made it official. She let go of life, piece by piece, while she was still in the midst of living it. One of the pieces she let go of was me. Not all of a sudden, not in any dramatic way, but progressively, incrementally, a slow, creeping chill that you don't feel until you're already half-frozen.

On Thanksgiving Day, a month and a half into my mother's stay in Oregon, I drive to the facility to pick her up and bring her home with me. I've been cooking since early morning: a big bird, home-made cranberry sauce spiked with Grand Marnier, twice-baked potatoes, and the stuffing my mother always made in a huge mixing bowl, working it with her hands—day-old dill rye cut into croutons, crimini mushrooms, diced celery, sweet onions, and several heads of roasted garlic.

On the drive over, I realize just how scared I am to have her at my house. All of our visits have been out at the care facility where she is surrounded by other women in various stages of dementia. Her shuffling walk, the silhouette of diapers under polyester pants, the pale vacant eyes—they all seem normal at the facility. There I can console myself that she isn't the worst one. One of her housemates is a bag of bones in a wheelchair. Another appears to be catatonic; a third twitches uncontrollably. At the facility there are caregivers who have seen it all, and I find that comforting. I can take my cues from them.

But it will be different at my house. I tell myself I'm scared because of the kids, because I'm afraid she'll do something weird and spook them. But it's not the kids; it's me. She spooks *me,* a ghost of who she was. There's just enough the same about her that, if the light is right, or if she strikes a certain pose, or if I don't have my contact lenses in, I can forget that she is not the same at all. But then she moves or she says something, and the illusion disappears. She is an old woman acting crazy, a woman I don't know. This unnerves me, even at the facility, even when she is in her element. In my home, it will be far worse. Her paintings hang on the walls. My cookbook is full of her recipes. In the upstairs linen closet my fitted sheets are folded the way she taught me. Everywhere there is evidence of the woman who used to be. I do not want to be confronted by the new evidence, the evidence of what she has become.

She has not been at the house since that first night she arrived, when she stayed over in the guest room and inexplicably made her own breakfast the next morning. Except for the Miracle of the Buttered Toast, I have no good memories of those eighteen or so hours and no desire to repeat the experience. But how can I have a family Thanksgiving dinner without her when she now lives less than ten miles away? Guilt is ultimately more powerful than fear.

She is dressed and ready to go when I arrive. I am relieved to see that the caregivers have not dressed her in polyester pull-on pants but rather in one of her good skirts, a warm brown wool with nubs of burnt orange and gold. She made it herself. I wonder if they noticed the personalized label sewn into the waistband. She's wearing a camel-colored, three-quarter-sleeve sweater that goes perfectly with the skirt and is fully accessorized with a thin gold-chain necklace, button earrings, and a bangle bracelet. It's wonderful to see her looking like she would have wanted to look. Then I notice the shoes. For thirty years my mother bought her shoes at only one store, Saks. She had an impossibly skinny foot, 7½ AAAA, and Saks was the only store she found that carried a variety of fashionable leather pumps in her size. On her feet today are a pair of old blue slip-ons, like deck shoes, and instead of stockings she has on knee-length hose meant for wearing under slacks. The skirt hits just at the wide dark band of elastic. From the knees up, my mother looks like a woman you'd see shopping at Saks. From the knees down, she looks like a bag lady.

I've prepped the kids—not Lizzie, who is just an infant, but the boys, ages six and eight. I've told them that grandma is "sick" and might "act a little funny." But I can see right away that they're oblivious. First of all, they don't really know grandma. They've seen her twice before when they were just toddlers but have no memory of those visits or the way she used to be before she got sick. Second, there's a new pirate Lego set under construction on the floor, so everything (and everyone) else is beside the point.

I install my mother in the rocking chair in the family room. The boys are playing at her feet. My husband and I are in the kitchen area, just a few feet away, staying busier than we need to be. My mother sits stiffly in the chair, not rocking. Her gaze is unfocused, her head turned away from me, in profile. I cook and talk. I don't know what I say, but I keep talking.

"Hey, lady," she yells. It takes a second before I realize she is talking to me. She sounds like Jerry Lewis doing one of his old routines: "Lay-dee! . . . oh, Lay-dee!" My husband and I look at each other, burst out laughing, and then feel weird and guilty about it. At least I do.

"Hey lady," she calls again. She has absolutely no idea who I am. "I'm thirsty," she says. I bring her a glass of water.

"Hey, lady," she says a few minutes later. "I'm cold." I get a fleece throw from the couch and lay it across her lap. At dinner, I sit next to her, cut up her food in bite-sized pieces, and put her fork in her hand. She eats everything.

14

Three times yesterday Susan reminded me about the party. Then, on my way out the door after a particularly grueling shift—nothing out of the ordinary, just plenty of it—she offered to call me at home this morning in case I needed an extra reminder. I had to laugh. "I got it," I told her. "Party. Tomorrow night. You can stop cueing me now." Cueing is a strategy we use with residents whose memory is muddled but not yet entirely erased. These residents need reminders to accomplish simple tasks—brushing teeth, putting on shoes—but they also want to feel as independent as possible. If we take over the task for them, we take away their independence. If we remind them too insistently, we erode their self-confidence. So we cue them with a gentle prompt, the subtext of which is *you probably would remember this anyway, but . . .* It's the way you'd remind your spouse to pick up a quart of milk on the way home. It's all in the tone of voice, in the offhand manner, subtleties that are absolutely not lost on these residents.

The dark humor that flows under this place like a subterranean stream is that all of us here—residents and employees alike—are losing our memories. Brooke, the twentysomething administrator, jokes about it when she blanks on the name of a family member of one of the residents. Jasmine jokes about it when she forgets she's left a load of laundry in the washer. Susan jokes about it every time she misplaces a pen or can't remember if the pet therapy lady said she would be bringing a dog or a goat that morning. Like so many jokes, it's masked fear. When you spend your days around people with this disease, despite the amazing moments and the times you feel like Mother Teresa on meth, the mantra that runs through your head is: *not me not me not me please not me*. We're scared, so we make jokes.

I give Susan a hard time about the cueing, but I don't think she's peppering me with multiple reminders about the party because she thinks I'll forget. I just think she's nervous. This party, billed as Hawaiian Night, is important to her and to strengthening her suddenly tenuous position at Maplewood. Susan has recently been getting signals from Corporate that her job as Life Enhancement Director is not highly valued. She now has to fight for every penny in her already skimpy activities budget, and just last week the powers that be took away her little office next to Brooke's and converted it into a records room. Now Susan works out of an empty bedroom in neighborhood 1. As soon as there is a paying resident for that room, she'll be moved again, to another vacant room, assuming there is one.

Unlike the cooks, the housekeepers, the RAs, the Med Aides, and the administrators, Susan is not involved in the delivery or management of basic services. What she does—plan and direct activities—is apparently considered nonessential, the "value-added," and thus expendable, component here. This just isn't true. If it were not for the activities, the music, the visiting animals, the field trips, the parties, Maplewood, for all its comfortable furnishings and sunny skylights and pretty parakeets in cages, would be a grim place indeed. There is more to life—even life with Alzheimer's—than a dry diaper and a hot meal. Susan's activities create their own kind of energy. They are, I think, both an anchor to reality for the people who live here and an escape from institutional boredom. The music, especially, seems to connect with so many of the residents, even the late-stagers.

Nevertheless, Susan finds herself marginalized at Maplewood, forced to prove and re-prove her own worth and the worth of her programs. That's why Hawaiian Night is so important to her. It will showcase her organizational prowess, her sense of fun, and, most important, her centrality to the lives of those who live here. If she can put on a good show, if she can attract a lot of family members and show them how much Maplewood cares, she strengthens her position here. Corporate might then see her not as an extraneous expense but as part of ongoing public relations efforts to keep paying customers happy. Family members, the ones who are footing the bills, will see that the check they write each month is buying more than custodial care.

As it turns out, Susan's worries about Hawaiian Night are groundless. That's clear the moment I walk into the atrium that evening and see the crowd. The turnout, Susan's main concern, is great. Of course all the residents are here, sitting in chairs placed around the perimeter of the large room, but so are scores of family members, including a number of people I've never seen here before. Elderly spouses, midlife children and grand-children, from infants to teens (teens being the only ones who look distinctly unhappy), flank the residents, many of whom are dressed in eye-popping flowered shirts and big floral Hawaiian prints. The colors are stunning: crimson, chartreuse, turquoise, hot pink, egg yolk yellow. Where did these wild clothes come from? I dress these people every day. I know their closets as well as I know my own. I've never seen this stuff before. The prints and colors animate their faces. Their white hair looks brilliant, like snow in the sunshine. They are all wearing plastic leis and holding plastic cocktail glasses filled with pink-tinged ginger ale. Each glass has a little paper umbrella sticking out of it. Susan, in a muumuu, strolls the perimeter, beaming.

Set up on one side of the atrium is Jim Kelley's Blast from the Past, the septuagenarians who appear so often here that they might be considered Maplewood's house band. Tonight they are playing Lawrence Welk bubble music with an island twist. It's never possible to ascertain if Jim and crew are enjoying themselves. They *look* festive with their flowery shirts and plastic leis, but their expressions are blank; their body language, unspoken. They just play. They play like file clerks file. But the Maplewood audience is an easy crowd to please.

Here is Addie, looking happier than I've ever seen her, which is not to say that she is smiling, but only that she is not whimpering, and her eyes are not downcast. She is, in fact, actively looking around, a rarity in my experience. Sitting next to her, patting her hand, is a big white-haired, bearded fellow who looks like Papa Hemingway. He has Addie's deep blue eyes. And here is Pam, a daughter on one side, a son on the other, and two toddler grandchildren playing with Hot Wheels at her feet. Across the room I see Frances M., but I don't quite believe what I see. She is up dancing with Susan, stepping side to side in time to Jim Kelley's rendition of "Little Grass Shack." Frances's daughter once told me that her mother loved to dance. But I could never picture it. Frances always moved so stiffly and with such an odd gait, a scuffling shuffle, quick and graceless. To see her move to music is a revelation. When I go up to her a few minutes later, she is sitting calmly next to her daughter—again, a surprise. Frances M. does not sit calmly. She does not sit at all. I ask her if she is having a good time, and she looks at me and answers the question. Yes, she says, I am—a direct answer to a direct question. Her daughter is grinning. This is a good day for Frances.

The residents, most of them, are "engaged," as Susan calls it. They are moving their heads to the beat of the music. They are tapping their toes. They are eating forkfuls of Costco cake. Family members are smiling. This evening, this event, is a reprieve for them, an hour or two during which they can almost forget about Alzheimer's. The mood is festive, the residents alert. You have to look hard to see evidence of disease. You have to strain to see anything institutional. The gathering might almost be mistaken for an old-fashioned community social, the kind of party that still takes place in rural Grange halls.

I'm here as a partygoer not a caregiver, so I have no duties. I am free to take in the whole scene and enjoy Susan's little triumph. She deserves it. And I too forget for a moment that I am in an Alzheimer's care facility. But the moment passes. It passes when I see Rose walk into the atrium from her neighborhood. It's like I am watching a movie. The movie is in Technicolor, bright and brilliant, noisy, buoyant, and up-tempo. There is Eloise in her vermillion silk blouse and Hayes on Mabel's arm and Pam, her head bent over a squirming grandchild while another runs happily around the perimeter of the room waving a plastic spoon. Then, walking through this movie, entering this colorful and merry scene, is Rose. She is silent, slow, in black and white, a specter. She shuffles across the room, shoulders sloping, head hanging, eyes at half-mast. She doesn't see the people or hear the sounds. She is untouched, an actor in her own private movie. Watching her sends a shiver up my spine, and I have to look away. I notice that others look away too.

When I come into work two days later, I am greeted with several surprises. A "surprise" in the context of this place is rarely a good thing. It's true that when Old Frances rebounded from hospice status, that was a good surprise. But it may be the exception that proves the rule. There are no surprise recoveries from this disease, no spontaneous remissions. The lame do not walk again; the blind do not see. A surprise is often the news that a resident has fallen or died or, less ominously and more frequently, that someone on staff has quit. This time, however, one of the surprises, the first one I encounter, is actually a good one.

A star. I have a star.

Thumbtacked to the bulletin board outside the break room is a yellow construction paper star with my name on it. *Lauren— She cares!* is printed in black marker. I have been waiting for this moment since I started working here.

I teach at a university, and a few years back, after going through a long review process, I got a letter informing me that I had been granted tenure. I am more proud of this paper star than I was when I got that letter. I don't know who is responsible for the star or what specifically I might have done to earn it, and I don't care. I don't care that the star carries with it not a single benefit. I don't care that no one outside the Maplewood world—which includes my family and friends—can really understand how thrilled I am. Still, I wish I could call my husband right now and tell him. But, star employee that I am, I am still not allowed to make personal phone calls during work hours.

I encounter the next surprise the moment I walk into the neighborhood. The first room I must pass on the way to my kitchen-area command post is Frances M.'s. When I glance through the open doorway as I walk by, what I see doesn't register for a moment. Then I do a double-take. Frances M.'s room is completely empty—no furniture, no flowered drapes, no wall art, no Frances. *She's dead,* I think. *She was dancing two days ago, and now she's dead.* The noc-shift RA, a bleary-eyed, care-worn woman I've never seen before, is sitting at the kitchen counter. I need to tell her that I'm here so she can go clock out. I'm afraid to ask her about Frances M.—I don't want to confirm my fears—but I ask anyway.

"Frances?" The noc-shift lady is drawing a blank. "Oh, you mean 129? She moved out yesterday."

"Moved out?" I'm confused. "Where'd she go?" I am thinking now that she fell, and she's in the hospital or a rehab center.

"Over to another neighborhood, I think."

Two hours later, when the administrative staff shows up for work, I find out that Frances M. was, indeed, moved to another neighborhood, neighborhood 1. Brooke is matter-of-fact about it, but we both understand the move for what it is—a "demo-tion." Neighborhood 1 is Rose's turf, home to the late-stagers. Frances M. was moved because she is just too far gone to make it in neighborhood 3. Any of the neighborhood 3 RAs would say that Frances M. is the most delusional and unpredictable of the residents, but that's been true for a while. I'm betting the move was negotiated because of the middle-of-the-night shower inci-dent that caused Jane's fall.

I can't say that I'll miss Frances M.—she was a lot of work and generally unpleasant to be around—but I will miss her sweet-natured, perennially upbeat daughter. This move must be a blow to her. Whenever Frances M. was having one of her increasingly rare lucid days, her daughter was gleeful. "Isn't Mom having a great day?" she would ask me (rhetorically) three or four times during her hour-long visit. During the Hawaiian Party two days ago, when Frances was as clearheaded and alert as I'd ever seen her, her daughter looked positively joyous, as if she thought her mother had suddenly turned the corner. The fever had broken. She was going to recover. She was going to be *okay*. I wish it worked that way. Now the daughter will be visiting in neighborhood 1, a sobering place. In neighborhood 1, the few women who can walk, shuffle. In neighborhood 1, everyone is hand-fed. In neighborhood 1, there is no conversation.

When I go to wake Hayes that same morning, I get yet another surprise: he has been catheterized. I don't inspect the origin of the catheter—I'll have to work myself up to do that—but I do trace the long clear plastic tube that snakes down under his pajama pants and leads to a now quarter-filled bag. I will have to learn how and when to empty this, and how to keep the site around the catheter clean, which is the bad news. On the plus side, I won't have to toilet Hayes every two hours, which is huge. I probably spend almost an hour of my eight-hour shift just getting Hayes back and forth to the bathroom.

I start to think of all the things I can do with that found hour—sit and talk with Jane, polish Eloise's nails, get to know Pam a little better—and then I am ashamed of myself. I'm treating this like good news, but it is obviously bad news for Hayes and his family. The catheter signals a problem. Something is not working right. I check Hayes's service plan. Whenever there's a change in routine—a resident has become shaky and now needs to use a walker, a resident isn't eating well and now needs a liquid supplement—it gets recorded in the margins of the service plan. The service plans of those who have been here for a while are crowded with such notations, a piecemeal chronicle of their (few) ups and (many) downs.

The RAs are supposed to read the service plans of all their residents every week and initial and date them. Brooke checks to see that we do this, and leaves polite but insistent memos on the staff bulletin board if we don't. I think reading the plans weekly is a good idea, and I try to comply. I try to find the time. But it's not uncommon for an eight-hour shift to go by without the opportunity to sit down and read, or, for that matter, to sit down for any purpose. It is possible for a whole week to go by without finding the time, unless I read during one of my breaks or clock out and read on my own time. And so, occasionally, like pretty much everyone here—except, I am sure, Calm Guam Frances—I initial a sheet without first reading it.

Had I actually read Hayes's plan *last* week, I would have seen that his doctor was treating him with antibiotics for a urinary tract infection. Although I care for Hayes several times a week, I am not surprised that I didn't know about the infection. People with Alzheimer's feel pain, but they rarely have the words to express or describe it. Maybe they get crankier than usual or more restless, maybe their appetite lags or they wake up in the middle of the night. Maybe these changes mean something, and maybe they don't. When my father was caring for my mother, she contracted a urinary tract infection, and it was a bad one. She must have been in pain, too, but she never said anything, and the infection went undetected until a routine doctor's visit.

I am also not surprised that I didn't know Hayes was taking a new medication, in this case, an antibiotic. I should know, the RAs should know because medications can have side effects that show up in daily behavior, but that's not how things work here. How it works is this: doctors phone or fax medical orders to Maplewood's part-time nurse, who instructs the Med Aides. The Med Aide on duty makes the rounds through the neighborhoods once or twice a shift to hand out pills. The RAs, the frontline caregivers, are just not in the loop.

Part of me understands why. After all, the RA turnover rate is astronomical. Time spent training or educating an RA is often wasted, as the trained person is out the door in a matter of weeks. And the extra instruction would not be insignificant. With many of the residents on multiple meds with varying side effects depending on other meds, other diseases, weight, gender, and who knows what else, just learning enough to be useful in one or two cases could be overwhelming. It is also difficult to imagine creating yet another chore for RAs: keeping track of (which would mean writing down regularly) any observed problems that could be medication related. Still, it seems like a flaw in management design, leaving the primary caregivers ignorant.

Reading *this* week's plan, I see that Hayes's doctor inserted the catheter because the antibiotics weren't working. Poor Hayes. He probably was in pain from the infection and is now undoubtedly, as those in the medical world like to put it, "experiencing some discomfort" from the catheter.

Two mornings later, another surprise: I go into Jane's room at 7:00 a.m. to wake her for breakfast and find no Jane and an un-rumpled, un-slept-in bed. What could have happened? Jane was fine on my shift the day before yesterday. She had completely recovered from her fall in the bathroom. She was moving well again, not using the walker. She was taking her strolls around the facility. She was sitting and talking with Pam, eating well, making jokes, chirping at the birds, handing out Tootsie Rolls. Maybe her daughter came to take her on an overnight outing. That must be it.

A few hours later, talking with an RA who was working the adjoining neighborhood yesterday, the Med Aide, and Brooke, I piece together what happened. Mid-afternoon yesterday, Jane started feeling dizzy. Her movements became odd and jerky; her speech slurred. She didn't respond to her name. She didn't know where she was. The RA did just what we're told to do: she immediately walkie-talkied the Med Aide, who rushed over, saw something was very wrong, and called 911. Within minutes, the

EMTs arrived, and Jane was whisked away in an ambulance. The word is she has had a massive stroke. I wonder if I'll ever see her again.

It's early September now. The summer is over; my youngest two kids are back in school, and my husband keeps asking when I'm going to stop working at Maplewood. When I took the job, I thought I'd work two weeks, just enough to understand what caregivers do, just enough to feel the rhythm of the days lived by the residents. But it's been more than a month and a half now, and I'm still signing up for my share of day-shift hours. *Why?* My husband wants to know. *You've done enough,* he tells me. *You've got your star. It's time to get back to real life.*

But right now this *is* real life to me, this Maplewood world. I don't know when I will leave it, but I know it's not time yet. It's not just that I have more to learn. It's that I have more penance to do, much more. The better I get at this job, the more I find ways to connect with and enjoy the company of the people I care for, the more I realize how badly I blew it with my mother.

Even with two Ensures a day, even with hand-feeding, my mother is still losing weight. She's now below a hundred pounds. Her clothes hang on her, and her face is gaunt. She holds herself in a new, stiff way, her muscles always tense, her jaw permanently clenched. Sometimes, helping her get out of bed, I cannot get her to bend her knees. My father's HMO won't cover it, but I take her to a local doctor for a full examination. Just getting her out of the facility and into my car takes close to an hour. She takes tiny, mincing steps, stopping every two or three and freezing in place. When we finally get to my car, which is only a few yards from the front door of her house, I can't manage to get her in. She won't bend at the waist. She won't lift one leg and put it inside my car. I try to pick her up, but I can't. Finally, by a combination of coaxing and shoving, I get her seated. I am exhausted by the time we arrive at the doctor's office. Although I've spoken twice to the nurse and been assured we would not have to wait in the waiting room, in fact, we sit there for forty-five minutes before the doctor sees us. My mother gets stuck in one of her repeating verbal patterns. People try hard not to stare at us.

The doctor—I choose a woman because women physicians are better listeners, more nurturing, or so I've read—treats my mother like an inanimate object, and not even an interesting inanimate object. The examination takes less than ten minutes. The doctor looks at a point a few inches above my head when she talks. Maybe she has Parkinson's, the doctor tells me. I get a bill a few days later for $330.

15

I am working a bit less these days but spending as much time as ever at Maplewood. If I work only two days one week, I go in the other three anyway. When I'm working a shift, it's impossible to spend quiet, uninterrupted time with anyone. I am lucky if I get to sit for five minutes with Eloise. My conversations are always on the fly, as I dash to Hayes's room or race over to the laundry area, as I collect the dishes from lunch or set up chairs for an activity. But when I'm here and not working, I can sit at the dining room table and leaf through magazines with the ladies, or relax with them on a bench in the outside courtyard, or watch old movies together on the couch. There's a new man in the neighborhood who has brought with him a ten-thousand-item baseball card collection. I bet this new guy would love to show me his favorite cards. I'm no fan, but my father took me to Shea Stadium a few times to see the Mets—the name Ed Kranepool comes to mind—and I could probably fake it. When I come in on a day off, we can sit together. I doubt he's had an attentive audience in years.

On my days off at Maplewood I am also free to explore the other neighborhoods, see other RAs in action—for both educational and (okay, I'll admit) competitive reasons—and get to know other residents. Yesterday I spent a delightful morning in neighborhood 2 with two women who have become best buddies since they arrived at Maplewood, as strangers, within one week of each other. That was about a month ago.

Vivian is a pretty woman, petite with a full head of curly silver hair that she wears free and loose, a little out of control, like she just rushed in from a brisk walk outdoors. She has good skin, with lines and wrinkles in the places you'd expect but not crepey, not sallow, not hanging loose around the jowls. Her features are soft and delicate. Her chart says she is eighty-three, but she looks barely seventy. When I tell her this, she smiles, a little embarrassed but clearly pleased. She is oblivious to how good she looks and probably always has been, in that easy unassuming way some women have who are born just pretty enough. She moves well, although she moves slowly, more slowly than she needs to, because she's usually holding the hand of Muriel, her best friend, who is a shuffler.

Vivian is very patient with Muriel, who is also eighty-three but looks it, a little woman with wispy hair that doesn't quite cover her scalp. Muriel has a tremor that shows as a facial tic. But you're not really aware of the tic because she has somehow managed to coordinate the twitch of her muscles with a click of her tongue against her hard palate. The twitch and the click are simultaneous. She moves her head from side to side keeping time with the clicks, smiling faintly. She clicks every two seconds, steady and predictable, like a metronome.

Why this doesn't drive Vivian crazy I don't know. But when I see that it doesn't, it makes me reevaluate my reaction. Repetitive behavior is a particularly tough one for me because of my mother, because of the way she used to get stuck in a verbal loop, repeating, repeating, repeating the same phrases. But Muriel is not my mother. I decide to follow Vivian's example and make peace with the clicks. I decide to look at the clicks in a new way. They are not irritating and annoying. They are instead a creative use of the spontaneous and unbidden energy that comes from Muriel's twitching facial muscles. I admire Muriel's inventiveness. I think of the clicks as music. Once or twice during the morning I even find myself clicking along.

Muriel is fluttery and clicky, but Vivian is utterly composed. Unless she is talking—her language is quite fluent—she sits quiet and still, hands folded on her lap. There is nothing listless or lifeless to this pose. There is, it seems to me, a deep sense of calm. I find this astonishing because, as it becomes obvious to me, Vivian is quite aware that she suffers significant memory loss. I have heard distressing stories about people in the early stages of Alzheimer's, people in that limbo between health and illness. Their memories are failing, but the fog has not yet enveloped them. They know something is wrong, but they can't do anything about it. I have heard that this is the very toughest time for people with the disease. Some days it seems Eloise is stuck in this limbo, that her agitation comes from the disquieting sense that something, but she doesn't know what, is just not what it should be. Vivian, however, doesn't seem to be struggling with this.

I ask her how she spends her days here. We are sitting around one of the dining room tables in neighborhood 2, she, Muriel, and I, drinking cups of tepid Lipton tea. Vivian thinks about the question for a moment.

"Let's see . . . what did we do yesterday?" she says aloud. "Muriel," she says, leaning over the table toward her friend, "what did we do yesterday?" Muriel smiles and clicks her tongue. Her gaze is unfocused. "We went out on the bus, didn't we?" Vivian says. Muriel clicks. "But what did we see? I wonder what we went out to see." She is looking over at Muriel. Muriel clicks, then looks her in the eyes and squints hard.

"I just can't understand what you're saying," Muriel says sweetly, in between clicks.

"Well, we had a good time. I know that," says Vivian. "I don't remember what we did," she tells me, smiling and shaking her head, "but that doesn't matter. It was sure fun while it was happening."

This morning, driving across town to Maplewood on another one of my days off, I think I'll visit with Vivian and Muriel again. Instead, when I walk in the front door, go through the lobby, and buzz myself into the facility, I make a beeline for Rose's neighborhood. I'm scared of what I'll see, but I am drawn there, in that weird and less than savory way people are drawn to bad things. It's that fascination with the macabre that makes drivers slow down on the highway to get a glimpse of an accident, or draws a crowd to a building to see if the person on the ledge will jump. (At least this happens in movies.) What is that instinct? It can't just be ghoulish curiosity, at least not all the time for everyone. I think part of it is testing yourself. *Am I strong enough to look this bad thing in the eye?* Part of it may be facing your own fears. *That could be me bloody by the side of the road.* And part of it is wanting–not wanting to know the worst. *Take a look. That's what death looks like.* I'm not sure which of these, if any, motivates me today. All I know is that I can't keep averting my eyes every time I see Rose.

Neighborhood 1—home to the end-stagers—is very, very quiet. I remember Jasmine telling me about the silence. On one of our first real days of work here, after training, she was temporarily assigned to this neighborhood. I saw her at lunch break, and her big eyes looked haunted.

"If this is what it's like, I won't be able to take it," she said. "It's *Night of the Living Dead* over there."

"You get used to it," one of the veteran RAs ("veteran" as in on the job for three months) told her. She told Jasmine that some RAs actually like working neighborhood 1 because "no one gives you any trouble."

Walking through neighborhood 1 this morning, I see what she means. Just about everyone is dozing. Three women are in their rooms curled up, fully dressed, on top of their made beds. The rest are out in the common area, slumped at the dining room table or caved in, chin-to-chest on couches and chairs in the living room. Their mouths hang open. I recognize one of the women. Her name is Florence, and back before I started working here, when I was just observing, I spent some time with her. She was in neighborhood 4 then, a pleasant, easily confused woman who had been a pianist and piano teacher all her working life. She didn't know where she was, and she had trouble dressing herself, but if you guided her over to the upright piano in neighborhood 3, where all the entertainment takes place, and sat her down, her hands remembered what her brain forgot. She was good. Now, a year later, Florence is in neighborhood 1, demoted like Frances M. was demoted. Florence is asleep in a chair, both knees drawn up to her chest, her wrists bent inward, awkward and frozen, like the hands of a quadriplegic. She looks too uncomfortable to be asleep, but I listen to her soft, even breathing, and I see her eyes move fast, side to side, under the lids. She is dreaming.

The only one not asleep right now, at ten in the morning, is an old lady everyone calls Grams. She's a tiny lady with sharp little bird eyes and straight white hair that sticks up all over, punklike. She is padding noiselessly across the carpet in her clean white tennis shoes, shoes so clean and so white that you know they've never been outside Maplewood. Grams has a dust rag in her hands. She stops at one of the dining room tables and sweeps the cloth back and forth, back and forth across the already clean surface. Then she sees something on the carpet under one of the chairs, maybe a piece of old food, and she stoops down to pick it up. She is very limber. While picking up whatever was down there, she notices dust on the legs of the chair and starts dusting. The RA says Grams does this all day—cleans and dusts and wipes, folds laundry, anybody's laundry, rinses out coffee cups in the sink. She rarely talks. She just works.

I watch her for a while and then go to sit on one of the couches in the living room in a space between Martha and Rose. Martha is a broad-shouldered lady with immense brown eyes that rarely stay open for more than a few minutes at a time. She is boxy, bulky, and silent, like an unplugged appliance. Next to her, Rose, stoop-shouldered and disheveled, looks smaller than she is. When I sit down, I wake them both. They look straight ahead but don't seem to notice what's playing on the TV screen just ten feet away. It's *My Fair Lady*, the 1964 musical starring Audrey Hepburn. Each neighborhood has a library of movies, old TV shows, and documentaries, everything from *Singin' in the Rain* to *I Love Lucy* to Australian travelogues. In my neighborhood, people sometimes actually watch this stuff. Here the RA probably puts in a video to keep from going nuts.

I have wonderful memories of *My Fair Lady*, the stage show, not the movie. It was the first Broadway play my mother took me to. She wore a black Persian lamb coat with a high collar and Arpège by Lanvin dabbed behind her ears. We had loge seats, second row. She flirted with the orchestra conductor during intermission. I was so proud of her.

"I just love this movie," I tell Martha and Rose. I hear how falsely cheery my voice sounds, but I'm the only one listening. Martha has already fallen asleep again. Rose is awake but sits inert, trancelike, unresponsive. We sit like this, silent, Martha dozing, Rose looking down at the floor, me staring at the TV screen thinking about my mother. Then, during one of the musical numbers, I notice that Rose is tapping her foot. She isn't watching the movie or seeming to pay attention, but she is keeping perfect time. During the next number, she keeps the beat by gently slapping her hand on her thigh.

The neighborhood RA is leaning over the couch, watching us. "Why don't you ask her to dance?" she says to me. She says it so matter-of-factly—no archness, no undertone of *wouldn't that just be so sweet?*—that dancing with Rose seems like a perfectly reasonable thing to do.

"Shall we?" I ask her, before I overthink the moment. She doesn't respond. I grab her hands and pull her up gently. She doesn't resist, but she doesn't help either. She stands in front of me, shoulders slumped, head down. I move closer, take one of her hands and position it on my shoulder, grab the other and hold it. She doesn't smell good. I put my arm around her waist, just above the elastic strip of her Depends. We hold on to each other like girls at a middle school dance. Eliza Dolittle has just launched into "I Could Have Danced All Night."

I press Rose's back with the palm of my hand and take the lead. I have so often seen her wander the neighborhoods of Maplewood, heavy-limbed and shuffling, an old, old woman at age sixty-eight, that I am amazed to discover that she can be light on her feet. She is—astonishingly—graceful as we start to waltz. I am not so graceful. I keep count in my head (the wrong count)—*one,* two, three, *one,* two, three—and sneak looks around the room to see who might be watching me make a fool of myself. The least of my concerns is that we are waltzing to a 4/4 beat.

Martha is sleeping on the couch. Florence is still scrunched uncomfortably in one of the big chairs, dozing. Grams is scrubbing the kitchen counter with a dry sponge. The RA has disappeared into someone's room. It's just Rose and me, Rose and me and the music that once thrilled me from the second row of the Mark Hellinger Theater. Rose is a good dancer. I stop counting to myself. I close my eyes and let her lead.

16

I'm in Hayes's room emptying his urine bag. This catheter thing is not working out well. It's true that I no longer have to toilet Hayes every two hours, which is great, and emptying the bag is really no big deal if you don't think too hard about what you're doing. But there's a problem I didn't anticipate: Hayes is in a constant and elevated state of curiosity about the tubing he sees emerging from his pants leg and looping over the side rail of his wheelchair.

I must admit, it *is* a pretty interesting sight when his pee is ever-so-slowly meandering through the clear plastic hose into the bag. *What is that? Where does it come from?* I imagine Hayes is thinking. Whatever he's thinking, he spends a lot of time plucking at the tubing, playing with it, pulling at it. In the past two days, he has managed to detach it from the bag more than a dozen times. His unending fascination with the apparatus is, in itself, fascinating. He must be mystified and curious day after day—it's now been more than a week—because he has virtually no short-term memory. Every time he looks down and sees the tube it's like the first time. *What is that? How does that work?* Hayes is ever the engineer.

Today when I'm in his room, he starts to talk to himself. It is not a muttering soliloquy but an actual conversation.

"I want to go home," Hayes says. Other residents say this. Eloise threw a fit about it just a while back, and a lady from neighborhood 4—one of the women involved in the "Old and the Restless" soap opera over there—is always stopping to tell me that she's packing to go home the very next day. But I've never heard this from Hayes. I think of him as completely acclimated to Maplewood, oblivious to any other life. He has been here for almost two years.

"Well, you can't go home," Hayes says, answering himself.

"How long do I have to stay here?"

"You have to stay here for the rest of your life."

"But that's not fair." Hayes's tone is not bitter, indignant, or even wistful. He's just making a statement.

"No, it isn't fair. But that's the way it is."

I feel like I should say something, standing, here in Hayes's bathroom eavesdropping on him talking to himself. But maybe there is nothing to say.

These past few weeks we've all been increasingly concerned about Hayes. The catheterization was one thing, but there's something else going on that's even more troubling. Maybe two weeks ago the decision was made to start pureeing all of Hayes's food. He was no longer able to eat whole food, even when we diced it in small pieces. He wasn't chewing. He wasn't swallowing. And so he wasn't eating. Now the kitchen is sending tall plastic glasses of hot liquefied food for Hayes's meals. However unappetizing Maplewood food sometimes looks, it looks far worse after it has been blender-whipped for sixty seconds. Imagine a pork chop and green bean smoothie.

But pureeing the food is not working either. When I try to feed it to Hayes, he rears back his head and won't open his mouth. I try to wedge the spoon in between his clenched teeth, but I can't. Look at me, Hayes, I say, and I open my mouth very wide. Do this. He does, and I shovel a spoonful of pureed whatever in his mouth. But it just lies there. Swallow, I say. I point to my throat. I swallow an exaggerated swallow. He looks bewildered. Then he starts spitting out the food. Hayes has always been a spitter, but before it was only after he had chewed, back when he was chewing, and found a little piece of gristly meat or fibrous vegetable. Now he's spitting liquid food. What he isn't spitting is remaining pooled in his mouth.

A slender fellow, he is now very skinny. His legs are all bone. Although he doesn't expend much energy—he is either sleeping or dozing close to eighteen hours a day—he can't afford to go very long without taking in some calories. Maplewood's nurse, after conferring with Hayes's doctor, makes the decision to stop trying pureed food. Maybe it's not smooth enough. Now we'll just go with Ensure shakes. He's always liked the chocolate flavor, and they're high in calories and have added vitamins. A few weeks ago he drank two entire cans of Ensure for me in one afternoon, smacking his lips and commenting often about how good the chocolate tasted.

But now when I place the cup to his lips and tilt it back so the liquid flows into his mouth, he does not swallow. The liquid pools in his mouth until it dribbles down his chin. We're all brainstorming solutions, Jasmine and me, Susan, Brooke, the nurse, Hayes's daughter Jennie, the cook. Maybe if we tweaked his taste buds. The kitchen tries fruit shakes—strawberry, peach, blueberry—with and without yogurt. Still he doesn't swallow. I try spoonfeeding him. I try a straw, but Hayes has forgotten what a straw is for. We are running out of ideas. We are not a medical facility. We can't feed him intravenously.

This inability to swallow is affecting not only his meals but also his meds. Until two weeks ago, the Med Aides gave Hayes his medication like everyone here: pills placed in the palm of the hand, glass of juice to wash them down. When Hayes first began having trouble swallowing, the Med Aides started mashing his pills and mixing them with a spoonful of applesauce or chocolate pudding. A few weeks ago, even last week, this strategy worked pretty well. Now it doesn't because he's not swallowing. It no longer works to cue him to swallow, to tell him to swallow, to show him, by exaggerated gesture, what swallowing is. Sandy, the day-shift Med Aide, has now taken to stroking his throat with gentle downward motions hoping to stimulate the esophageal muscles. Sometimes she manages to get the pills down this way, but most often the medicated pudding or applesauce sits in his mouth until he spits it out.

I remember what a hospice nurse once told me about eating and swallowing and the end of life. She had seen dozens of people die, scores, maybe hundreds. She didn't count. Some had Alzheimer's; many did not. She visited them in the weeks and days and hours before they died, and she was there at the moment itself. I said: What a sad job. How very stressful. How did she stand it? She smiled. It wasn't a beatific, patron-saint-of-the-deathbed smile, but rather a plain, down-to-earth middle-aged-woman's smile. She said the job was a privilege, that it was the best job she'd ever had.

I was asking her about eating and swallowing because back then, my mother was beginning to have significant problems. These problems made sense to me from a medical point of view.

I figured it was part of the awful progression of the disease. First the plaques and tangles clogged the brain enough to impair memory and judgment, then cognition and communication and, finally, the ability to remember and execute the simplest of tasks like eating and swallowing.

But this hospice nurse had another take on it. Not that she argued with the physiological progression, not that she in any way doubted that plaques and tangles so mucked up the brain that it began to malfunction. But being around dying people, experiencing the ebb of the life force, she had a humanistic, holistic, nonclinical view of death. The body, she told me, knows it is dying. And it knows it does not need to take in nourishment for this task. In fact, if nourishment is taken, then energy is diverted. The body will have to digest the food, carry it through the stomach, small intestines, large intestines, carry nourishment to the cells, excrete the waste. The liver will be involved, the pancreas, the gallbladder. And for what? For staying alive. That's why she believes a person in the process of dying refuses food, stops chewing, stops swallowing. It has little to do with Alzheimer's.

I don't know what doctors would think of this explanation, but it makes deep and perfect sense to me. It taps into what we, steeped in Western medicine, seem to be slowly relearning: the wisdom of the body. It is interesting, and comforting, to think of death as the silent, purposeful act of a wise and ailing body, not a jarring event but a transition, a process, almost a routine, commonsense and familiar, like walking through the house at night, checking on the kids, locking the doors, and turning off the lights before you go to sleep.

Two weeks ago, I was getting Hayes out of bed every morning. He was standing with his walker and moving slowly to the bathroom, walking. I sat him in his wheelchair or in his big blue chair by the window. He made the usual nuisance of himself, forever calling for someone to scratch his back. He listened to music. He dozed. Now he doesn't want to get out of bed at all. He says he's too tired. Of course he is too tired. He has no energy coming in, no energy reserves. His body is beginning to shut down.

Brooke has a long, painful meeting with Jennie, Hayes's daughter. Clearly, it's time to do something else for Hayes. Maplewood can no longer care for him in the way he now needs to be cared for. One option is the hospital. If he goes there, and if the family chooses, he would receive aggressive therapy. He could get intravenous glucose. He could get intravenous meds. He could be hooked up to monitors. If he stopped breathing, they could put in a trache tube and bag him. If his heart stopped beating, they could do CPR, put paddles on his chest, shock him back to life. His body could be kept alive by machines. That's what end-of-life has become for many people, sometimes because family members are not prepared to see their loved one die, sometimes because they've seen too many doctor shows on TV and believe that medical miracles happen every day. "Heroic measures" these all-out, end-of-life efforts are sometimes called. I wonder who the hero is here: The doctors who don't want to get sued for failing to do everything possible to sustain life? The hospitals that have invested millions in machinery and high-tech gadgetry and need to get back their investment? Our culture that excludes illness and dying and death from the business of life? I don't see any heroes. I don't want Hayes to go to the hospital.

And neither, it turns out, does Jennie, his daughter. She is not sure what she wants, but it's not that. More important, she's not sure, no one is quite sure, that this is Hayes's endgame. After all, Old Frances also stopped eating and didn't want to be roused from bed and was put on deathwatch, and she came back. Brooke and Jennie decide to confer with the hospice service based at the local hospital. It may be that Hayes's life is unsustainable, that he is ready to die, and that, just as important, his children are ready to let him go. This is something the hospice people can help determine. They can also offer a plan that treats Hayes with dignity and respect, a blueprint for the process of dying that can take place here at Maplewood, here in Hayes's room. Brooke makes the call on Tuesday. The first appointment she can get is Friday. In the meantime, we RAs continue to wake Hayes every morning. Sometimes, despite his objections, we get him up and dressed, and plant him in his chair. Sometimes he seems so frail, and every touch makes him wince, that we leave him be. We offer fruit shakes and chocolate Ensures, whole milk and juice. Occasionally he manages to swallow the tiniest sip. We play music for him. He sleeps. Every day he is weaker. Every day he talks less.

Thursday afternoons the consulting geriatric nurse practitioner comes to Maplewood to evaluate residents. The nurse examines Hayes and rules out the possibility of an Old Frances–style rebound. This really is it for Hayes, she says. Then she spends the rest of the afternoon closeted with Jennie, Brooke, and Christine, the Care Coordinator, so they can jointly hammer out an end-of-life plan. What does the family want for Hayes? What *exactly* do they want? The plan must be precise and detailed, clinical in language but caring in nature. They work through it, category by category. Nourishment: we are to keep offering shakes and Ensures, but if Hayes is not swallowing, we are to discontinue. There will be no pushing of fluids. Medication: the determination is made to "DC" (discontinue) most of Hayes's meds. The only ones he'll be offered are those necessary for his physical comfort, his thyroid pills and a stool softener.

He will also start getting regularly scheduled doses of Roxinol, liquid morphine, with orders to give him more if needed. This is probably the most common end-of-life medication, a gentle elixir that both relaxes muscle tension and dulls pain. And it doesn't need to be swallowed. Administered by medicine dropper either under the tongue or between cheek and gum, it enters the blood stream quickly through the mucous membranes. The plan also spells out the details of what is called "comfort care," the things we RAs and the family will do for Hayes: keeping him clean and warm, shifting his position to relieve pressure points, arranging pillows and pads, checking his skin and applying lotion, putting Vaseline on his lips, swabbing the inside of his mouth to keep it moist.

After the meeting, Jennie and Mabel, Hayes's wife, spend time with him in his room. We have roused him from his bed, and he sits in his chair by the window dressed in his usual preppy outfit—plaid shirt under V-neck cotton sweater, khakis. The clothes now look two sizes too big for him. Sandy, the Med Aide, comes in with his pills, which are mashed and mixed with chocolate pudding.

"Look, Dad," says Jennie. "Look, Dad. It's chocolate. Chocolate is your favorite thing."

"Your favorite thing next to Mabel," Sandy adds. Mabel, who is sitting on a chair next to Hayes, doesn't hear the remark. But Hayes does.

"Mabel," he says. "Mabel, Mabel, strong and able." She hears him. He's recited that little ditty for as long as she can remember. She stretches out her arm to touch him.

On Friday, the hospice nurse and social worker arrive at Maplewood. They review Hayes's medical records, noting the vital signs, the behavior, the eating habits, his medications. All have been faithfully recorded by the Med Aides and the RAs. They read the comm logs, the anecdotal accounts we RAs keep about the residents. What they see, what anyone can see, is that

Hayes's health has been going through significant changes, none of which are for the better. He has been losing ground every week, and now, it seems, every day. The nurse and the social worker meet with Jennie and two of her sisters. It is decided that Hayes is "appropriate" for hospice, which is to say that Hayes is dying, and that the family has decided there will be no heroic efforts to sustain his life.

The hospice workers go over the plan Jennie and the geriatric nurse detailed yesterday to make sure it expresses the wishes of the family. They arrange to have a hospital bed set up in Hayes's room. The family also wants someone with him, in his room, through the night, not just the noc-shift RA checking on him every hour or so, not just the Med Aide making her rounds, but someone sitting by his bedside. Jennie contracts with an elder-care service to send a private caregiver. She will start that night, Friday, to sit with Hayes. Everything is now in place.

The family stays late into the afternoon, through dinner—which Hayes is unable to eat—and into the evening. They are trying to get used to this change, not just the change in their father but the change in themselves, their acknowledgment that Hayes is going, their acceptance of it. Jasmine, who is on duty tonight, transfers Hayes back to his bed, the bed with soft flannel sheets washed in Ivory Snow. Hayes's body is all sharp angles now, his bones and joints visible beneath his papery skin. The private caregiver arrives, but still Jennie doesn't leave. Brooke has set up one of the unoccupied bedrooms in the neighborhood so that Jennie and others in her family have a private place to sit or talk or rest or sleep.

On Saturday, the family is back, Mabel and five of Hayes's children. He is in bed. He sleeps almost all the time. His handsome face is a skull loosely wrapped in parchment. He does not open his eyes.

In the early afternoon, he begins to run a fever. Sandy, the Med Aide, is keeping a close watch. The fever continues to rise, hour by hour. Hayes has become completely unresponsive. If he is not technically in a coma, he is certainly experiencing something deeper and more significant than sleep.

Is he busy dying? Is he somewhere in between here and there? I think of the Dylan lyric "He who is not busy being born is busy dying." So we are all busy dying, not just Hayes? I have a hard time with this idea, poetic as it is. After all, when we're healthy, or at least when our bodies are making an attempt to keep us alive, life is in a constant state of regeneration. We are, in fact, busy *living,* and it is a hectic, full-time business. Our bodies make 2 million new red blood cells every second. Our bodies make a new outer skin, all new cells, every twenty-seven days. We are a biochemical factory working 24/7, full employment, all shifts, busily manufacturing the parts we need to keep ourselves alive. As I look at Hayes's frail sleeping body, I need to hold on to the image of my own healthy body, my regenerating factory, as if this conjured image could ward off death, my death. As Hayes lets go of life, it seems I need to grasp it even more firmly. I want to shake him awake so I can thank him. Lying there, still and silent, this old man is forcing me to think about, as Douglas Adams wrote in *The Hitchhiker's Guide to the Galaxy,* "life, the universe and everything."

"How long?" Mabel, Hayes's wife, asks Sandy, the Med Aide. It's late afternoon now, and Mabel has been with Hayes since breakfast. Mabel has been with Hayes since FDR's first term. "How long does he have?" Sandy demurs. She is not a nurse. She cannot make that determination. But she knows Mabel needs to hear something.

"Maybe a couple of hours," Sandy says. "Maybe a couple of days."

Mabel is exhausted and so is Jennie. Still, they keep vigil, cooling Hayes's feverish forehead with damp washcloths, putting ice chips between his dry lips. They stay several hours more. When they finally leave, mid-evening, they make Sandy promise to call if there is any change at all. The private caregiver remains.

Sandy comes in every hour to check on Hayes and to reposition him in the bed. He looks peaceful, she thinks. He looks comfortable. But at 10:00 p.m., her final check before going off shift, Sandy notices a change in Hayes's breathing. He is panting softly, in quick shallow breaths, from the top of his chest. Then she hears a hoarse, congested sound coming from his throat. But Hayes is not gasping for air. He is not struggling. His face is in repose. He is immobile, comatose. She's heard that sound before, that guttural groan. Sandy hurries to call Jennie. Come back, she tells her. It's time.

Jennie quickly makes the phone calls. Within an hour, Mabel, Jennie, and four of Hayes's other children are in his room. He is curled in a fetal position on his right side, the way he always sleeps. He is wearing sky blue pajamas. He is surrounded by pillows. He is surrounded by family. At 12:25 a.m. he stops breathing.

17

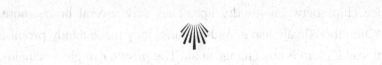

Jane is back! There she is, sitting at the dining room table, holding a glass of juice in her hand, her broad face creased with a smile. Her eyes are bright; her color is good. She is talking to Pam about how much she missed the parakeets while she was away. She makes it sound as if she'd gone on holiday, a cruise, maybe. In fact, she spent five days in the hospital and two weeks in a rehab facility. Her return—especially in such fine fettle—has me almost believing in miracles. I go over and hug her and make such a big deal that Jane starts to blush and tells me to cut it out.

The good news, and the reason she's back here laughing and talking and being her own Jane-self, is that she apparently did not suffer the massive stroke originally feared. She had, instead, a stroke lite, a TIA, which stands for transient ischemic attack. A TIA can look like a stroke—the same symptoms of difficulty speaking, unusual behavior, vertigo, weakness, numbness—but it's more like a rehearsal for one. A TIA is a brief and temporary interruption of blood flow to the brain caused by a clot in an artery. *Temporary* is the operative word. Because the blood flow stops for only a short time, there is often no significant permanent damage.

But that's not what Jane's daughter and son-in-law thought when they rushed to the hospital after getting the distress call from Maplewood three weeks ago. Jane looked bad, very bad. Her eyes were cloudy and unfocused. She couldn't stand. She could barely speak. Although doctors soon ruled out a stroke and made the new TIA diagnosis, and although her symptoms abated, things still did not look good. Almost a week after what was termed "the event," Jane was still disoriented. Her short-term memory seemed almost nonexistent. She repeatedly asked where she was and what had happened, and it didn't matter how many times her daughter or son-in-law or the nurses told her, nothing registered. But her physical symptoms were gone, and she was in no pain. There was nothing more the hospital could do for her.

Her daughter and son-in-law found a spot for her at a local rehab facility, a somber place, a sort of holding bin for discharged but still clearly dysfunctional elderly patients. Jane, like the other people there, had survived a medical crisis. These folks were not sick enough to stay in the hospital—their insurance wouldn't have paid for it anyway—but not healthy enough to go back home or to assisted living or a place like Maplewood. So they came to an old people's halfway house like the one Jane's family found for her. They're called rehabilitation facilities, but in truth, the rehab efforts are relatively minor, unless the family hires a physical therapist to come in.

Jane had the middle bed in a triple room with a loquacious neighbor on one side and a bed-bound woman who moaned all day on the other. The staff did get her up and moving, walking every day. At first she shuffled, leaning heavily on her walker.

But as her legs got stronger, she began to move like the Jane of old, using the walker only for balance. That was the good news. The bad news was that Jane seemed no less disoriented than she had been in the hospital. She recognized her family, but she still didn't know where she was or why. Her short-term memory was as bad as it had been a day after the ministroke. Her daughter and son-in-law talked to her about Maplewood, about her friends there, about her daily routines and how she would soon be returning to them. She remembered nothing. She retained nothing. Her daughter figured that the TIA on top of the Alzheimer's had pretty much zapped Jane's brain.

After two weeks, the rehab place could do no more for her. When her son-in-law came to collect her, she was upset, confused, and agitated. He didn't tell her they were going to Maplewood because the name meant nothing to her. Instead, he said they would be "stopping off somewhere" to see a few of the people who had visited her during the past two weeks. He meant Brooke and Susan, both of whom had made several trips after work to check up on Jane. When Jane and her son-in-law arrived at Maplewood, there was not a glimmer of recognition from Jane. She had no idea who Brooke and Susan were.

The son-in-law walked her into the neighborhood. She recognized nothing. Pam came over to say hello. Marianne greeted her. Still nothing. He didn't know what to do. He was going to have to leave her here, but how could he? To her, this was a strange place. All these people were strangers. He unlocked the door to her room and tried to walk her in. She stood frozen in the doorway. Then, slowly, she rotated her head a full 180 degrees and took in the room: the twin bed with the satiny flowered bedspread, the chest of drawers with framed pictures and a small stack of books, the easy chair by the window, the TV with the vase on top.

"Thank God," she said. "I'm back home." And that was it. From that moment she was Jane again, which meant that neighborhood 3 could be neighborhood 3 again.

While Jane had been away, a new resident moved in, a big, shambling man named Larry. He moved into the room next to Jane's, the one Frances M. used to occupy before she was demoted out of here to neighborhood 1. Larry has big, thick glasses, ill-fitting upper and lower false teeth, and skin that hangs on him like a slipcover made for a bigger couch. His complexion is dead gray. He breathes quick and shallow, wheezing with both inhalation and exhalation. Before I do anything else, I grab the service plan notebook and speed-read Larry's file. I see that he has severe asthma, but he's not on oxygen or inhalation therapy. The chart says he can walk with a walker, but this is one of those ridiculously optimistic (or cost-saving) notations from the family. Larry can barely stand up. His legs can hardly hold the weight of his body, even when he leans heavily on the walker.

I'll have to get to know him, figure him out, see how he fits in here. I know this is what happens at eldercare facilities everywhere: change, readjustment, more change. The places are always in flux. Old residents leave, often feetfirst. New residents arrive to take their place, bringing with them new issues, new behaviors. In my own neighborhood within just a few months, Ella died, and her place was taken by another woman; the guy with the baseball card collection moved into a vacant room; Frances M. moved out; Jane left—and then returned; Larry moved in; and of course, Hayes died. We RAs have to get used to this, not just saying good-bye but also hello, learning the habits and foibles of new residents, what help they need, what they eat, whom to sit them next to, how to connect with them. The caregiver's job changes as the residents change, and the residents change often. But then, so do the caregivers. I've heard that the most intense kind of stress comes from change over which you have no control. On that basis, I'm guessing this job qualifies, in spades.

At lunch, I cut up Larry's food and stand by his side, spearing pieces of meat with the fork and laying it back on the plate for him to pick up. His hands shake so badly that he can barely maneuver the fork to his mouth. In his service plan it says he needs no assistance eating. I stand there and guide every forkful. When he is finally done—the guy does have a healthy appetite, even if nothing else about him is healthy—he announces he has to go to the bathroom, another activity for which he needs "no assistance." I pull back his chair and place the walker in front of him. His hands are so palsied that I have to take hold of them and position them on the walker for him. He can't pull himself up. I wrap my arms around his chest, bend my knees and lift. He weighs maybe 180 pounds. I know I'm crazy to be doing this by myself. But with only one Float serving four neighborhoods, I could wait for assistance for ten or fifteen minutes. And *now* is when Larry has to go to the bathroom, not ten or fifteen minutes from now.

I lift him from the chair to an upright position so that he is standing in front of his walker. It's not easy, but I can do it because I work out at a gym, I swim, I'm healthy. But I wonder how my coworkers manage to do this—the lifting, the bending, the literally miles and miles of walking each shift—day after day, week after week. Most of them, even those in their twenties, are in bad shape. Almost everyone smokes. Almost everyone is in high-stress mode every day, shuttling between the challenges of Maplewood and unpredictable, often chaotic home lives. They eat the kind of food that supersized Morgan Spurlock into ill health in less than thirty days—and they've been eating it for years. They've gone decades without seeing a doctor, a lifetime with no medical insurance. I continue to be astonished when I learn employees' ages around here: thirty-year-olds who look fifty, forty-five-year-olds who look like they could be the mother of most forty-five-year-olds I know.

I position Larry behind his walker and point him in the right direction. He walks step by labored step across the dining area and to the nearest bathroom. It takes almost five minutes for him to negotiate the twenty steps. He is wheezing and sweating. I am holding his walker with one hand and supporting him around the waist with the other. We have to stop after every step. I can't believe we're going to make it to the bathroom in time. Regardless of what it says in his service plan, this man needs a wheelchair. When we finally get over the threshold of the bathroom, Larry collapses, crumbling slowly to the linoleum floor. I see it happening in slow motion, hold on to his waist, position my body behind him, and guide him down. He is so heavy that he takes me down with him. But neither of us is hurt. I've buffered his fall, and somehow, miraculously, not injured myself in the process. Now I *do* need help.

Inez, the Med Aide on duty, answers my call on the walkie. You can get immediate help if it's an emergency. She'll be right over, she says. I sit on the floor behind Larry rubbing his back, waiting. I've worked only one shift before with Inez and barely know her, but when she arrives a minute later to help me get Larry up and on the toilet and immediately launches into a personal conversation, I am not surprised. Perhaps it's the physical intimacy of the job, or that in a pinch you really have to trust and depend on your coworkers even when they are strangers; maybe it's the stress of the job. Whatever it is, they sometimes blurt out personal things when you hardly know them. One woman I had never met who came out for her ten-minute break when I was just finishing mine told me her boyfriend beat her.

Another woman confided, as we both dumped our trash in the outside Dumpster, that she was on antidepressants. Lena regularly corners me—or anyone else she can get—to relate in detail the unsavory behavior of boyfriends, exes, and various sons-in-law.

Inez is a blocky, fiftyish woman with salt-and-pepper hair who looks weary and well worked. But she is strong enough to help me with Larry. I tell her Larry really needs a wheelchair. Could she see if whoever is paying for his care will spring for one? She says she'll write it in her report. Her husband, she tells me, is in a wheelchair. He has multiple sclerosis. She's driving him up to the VA Hospital in a few weeks to get another round of steroid treatments that may put him in temporary remission. Last year he had a heart attack. He hasn't worked in five years. Inez, at $7.25 an hour, is the family breadwinner.

The next day, I arrive at Maplewood just in time for the mandatory monthly staff meeting. The meeting day always coincides with payday—which is basically what gets people to come in, that and the threat that they can be fired if they miss the meeting. But the paycheck is really the motivator: it's what brings in the noc-shift workers who would rather be sleeping, the swing workers who don't have to report for another hour, and those, like me, who are on their day off. (For those on duty right now there is a separate mandatory meeting scheduled after their shift ends, which means they stay an hour later, off the clock, of course.) You come to the meeting, and Patty hands you your envelope, $290 a week before taxes if you've worked full-time. You can't wait for the check to be sent. You need the money now, today. It is my privileged position to not need the money at all. It has also been my privileged position to not have to attend these meetings until now.

But I choose to come today because I have something to contribute to the meeting. I want to bring up a few no-cost suggestions that I think will make the job a little more efficient, just minor things like labeling the residents' drawers so their clothes are easy to find and put away (like Hayes's daughter used to do) and standardizing where we put toiletries so we don't waste time looking. I assumed these staff meetings would provide opportunities for RAs to talk about issues that affect them, to bring up concerns, to make suggestions. But I am wrong. Apparently, these are the kind of meetings where the underlings sit and are talked at.

Susan, who is first on the agenda, launches into the importance of spending quality time with the residents, of engaging them in activities. Leaf through magazines with them, she tells us. Look at family scrapbooks with them. Ask them about the photographs in their rooms, the objects. Each one has a story. We cannot think of these people as just waiting around to die, Susan says. She's right, of course, but she's preaching to a tough crowd—twenty-five overworked women forced to come into Maplewood when they're not on duty. People squirm, check their watches, close their eyes for a moment. Susan is so involved in what she's saying that she doesn't see that no one is listening. For the second half hour of the meeting, a physical therapist lectures us on how to lift patients correctly, which we've all heard before and all pretty much ignore. Then, the meeting is over. No discussion, no new business, no questions or concerns.

After the meeting I overhear Brooke and the nurse talking about Rose. Things can change so quickly here. I haven't spent any time with Rose since our waltz in 4/4 time, but until recently I have seen her around. Just last week Rose was her usual ghostly self, haunting all the neighborhoods, shuffling who knows how many miles down hallways and into rooms. I hadn't seen her for the past few days but thought nothing of it. Now I hear that the day before yesterday she walked into the room of a new resident in her own neighborhood, a man named Bob whom I've never met. Rose always goes into other people's rooms. This is pretty much what she does all day. Most people ignore her—or her presence simply doesn't register. I used to walk into Hayes's room and find him happily listening to music in his chair with Rose curled up on his bed a few feet away.

But apparently, Bob is different. Bob is territorial, protective of the one place he can call his own, his bedroom here. As a newcomer, he is probably not settled in to the rhythm of the place, probably still edgy. At any rate, it seems that Bob saw Rose go into his room and went in after her. No one knows exactly what happened in the few seconds between that and when the neighborhood RA came in, but some kind of skirmish took place, and both Bob and Rose landed on the floor. The word is that Rose broke her hip, but that it's not a bad fracture, and they were able to put a pin in. Now she's at a rehab facility in the south part of town, just like the place Jane was in. Brooke isn't sure when Rose will be back. I find out the name and address of the place from Patty. I'll go by there later this afternoon, after I spend some quality time with Eloise and Jane, after I check in with that inseparable duo in neighborhood 2, Vivian and Muriel, the human metronome. I have a chance to do just what Susan told us she wants us do to while we are working—because I'm not working.

An hour and a half later, my visits complete, I am talking to Brooke in front of her office when Patty walks over and whispers something in Brooke's ear. I am close enough to hear it. A call has just come in: Rose is dead.

18

A week later, a gorgeous early fall afternoon, the sky cornflower blue and cloudless, I drive to a neighboring town to attend Rose's funeral. The funeral home is not one of those stately old full-of-character houses, like in *Six Feet Under*, but a window-less, one-story concrete building that could be mistaken for a machine shop or a plasma donation center. Inside, the "chapel" is arranged like a church, with rows of wooden pewlike benches facing what is supposed to be a pulpit but is really just a ply-wood podium. There is no stained glass, no paintings or statues or icons, no hint of the spiritual or the religious here.

In front is a table on which sit three potted plants, purple mums, three lit candles, and a framed photograph of Rose and her husband, probably from the early 1980s. Rose has a big, boxy face surrounded by an unattractive helmet of dark hair, too dark for the face, dyed probably. The woman in the photograph doesn't look much like the Rose I knew, except that maybe the expression is the same: grim and almost aggressively cheerless, as if she is daring anyone to give her something to smile about.

There's a CD player on the floor behind the podium. Oddly, a Norah Jones song is playing, her voice husky and sexy and wildly inappropriate. *Come away with me in the night.* Most of the benches are empty. I count twenty-two people here; none, except for me, from Maplewood.

The music plays; people sit silently, waiting for something to happen. Five minutes go by, ten, fifteen. I entertain myself by imagining that Rose is here right now. She is shuffling down the aisle, conscious of no one but herself, no, not even herself. She is picking up one of the pots of purple mums from the front table and carrying it away. She is picking up a lady's purse from the bench. Someone grabs her arm and tries to stop her, redirect her, attempts to extricate the purse from her grip. Rose has quite a grip. She will have none of it. She is totally, perfectly, obliviously who she is. When you're around her, you play by her rules. You've got to admire her for that.

Finally, the minister or pastor or whoever he is—he is not introduced nor does he introduce himself—walks up to the podium. He talks about Rose's life: how she married her high school sweetheart at sixteen, how they raised three daughters and a son, the great times they had going to drive-in movies or to the lake for waterskiing or skinny-dipping. How Rose's house was a center of activity for the neighborhood kids. How Rose was an avid gardener and a league bowler. How fun loving she was. What a playful spirit she had.

I'm working hard to wrap my mind around an image of Rose the Blithe Spirit, Rose the Jocular, when I hear him say that at Maplewood Rose was known as "the welcome lady" because she greeted everyone with a big smile. I wonder where he got *that?* The disconnect between the person being talked about and the person I knew is so complete that I feel momentarily disoriented. Maybe I walked into the wrong funeral. Maybe the minister is reading from the wrong set of notes. (The next day, I do a reality check with Susan. What was Rose like back when she first got here, I ask, back when she wasn't as far gone as the woman I knew? Was she fun loving? Did she greet everyone with a smile? Susan looks at me like I'm nuts. Susan, who has something good to say about everyone, who loves everyone, who loved Rose, tells me Rose was ill-tempered and contrary from the moment she arrived at Maplewood. Her home life before she got to Maplewood was—and here Susan pauses meaningfully—"very difficult.")

At the service, the minister is saying that Rose "sowed seeds of laughter and joy everywhere she went." Okay, I understand about not speaking ill of the dead. At my funeral I don't want someone going on about how bossy I was or how hard to please, taking time to comment on my many and varied faults and bad habits. But on the other hand, I don't want complete lies. I don't want the people sitting in the pews—and I'm sure they will be *legion*—rolling their eyes and shaking their heads. I look around the "chapel" surreptitiously to see how the audience is taking the minister's creative retelling of Rose's life, but the faces I can see are impassive masks.

The minister asks who would like to come forward with a remembrance of Rose. No one makes a move. I look up at the first bench and see that Rose's daughter, the only one Susan remembers ever having visited—and she did not visit often—is sitting with people I assume are her siblings. They are sitting motionless facing front. Their shoulders do not touch. They don't bend their heads to whisper, don't extend their arms to comfort each other. I wonder what lies at the heart of this family.

Who would like to say something about Rose, the minister asks again. I look around the room and try to imagine who these people are. There are a few older people, friends, I guess, and some younger couples—nieces and nephews? Grandchildren? The minister said that Rose had six grandchildren and two great-grandchildren, an unusual accomplishment given that she wasn't even seventy yet. My mother was Rose's age when her *first* grandson, my oldest son, was born. Of course, when you marry at sixteen as Rose did, your life has an altogether different chronology.

With four children and six grandchildren surely someone has a memory of Rose to share. A neighbor? A fellow bowler? What about those "seeds of laughter and joy"? No one comes forward. The silence is uncomfortable. The minister tries but fails to hide his surprise. He's just not sure what to do up there behind the plywood podium. I am tempted to go up and talk about the time Rose and I danced together. But I don't. I'm an outsider, an interloper at this funeral. It is not my place to offer a memory when Rose's own family is silent.

The minister waits a little longer, scans the pews, looks down, scans again. He is avoiding looking at the first bench where Rose's children are sitting. Finally, he starts in again. "God has prepared a place where Alzheimer's is cured and broken hips are mended," he says. "That's where Rose has gone to." I wonder if anyone is buying that. I wonder if there is comfort in those words. I hope so.

Back at Maplewood the next day, I am telling Nadine, the regular day shift RA in Rose's neighborhood, about the funeral. She is a big girl with pale, tired eyes and a soft voice. I've always liked her. "Some of the other RAs say that it's a relief that Rose is gone," she tells me. "But I miss her . . . I really do." She starts to cry. "The neighborhood is just not the same without her."

The weather changes suddenly. By the end of the week, the days are raw, foggy, and damp, the sky the color of cement. Friday is the kind of day that, even if you weren't going to a funeral, you'd feel funereal. But I *am* going to one, my second this week—Hayes's. The church is out River Road, which during the time Hayes raised his family here and operated his machine shop, was a quiet, winding rural road that passed through apple and filbert and berry orchards as it followed the curves of the Willamette River. Now it is more highway than street, four lanes of forty-five-miles-per-hour traffic that pass through housing developments and strip malls. Out where you can still see a bit of open land is the church, one of those sprawling complexes with a circular chapel that probably looked so hip in the mid-1970s that the congregation almost didn't fund it.

When I get there ten minutes early, the parking lot is full, and cars are pulling up on the grass. Inside, it is SRO, 150 people at least. In the chapel-in-the-round, a spirited elderly woman is seated at a piano banging out one of the songs Hayes loved, the one that goes, "When the red, red robin comes bob-bob-bobbin' along." I scan the room and count nine people from Maplewood. Brooke is here sitting near the family, and Susan is here with her husband, Scotty, a retired pastor who leads "spirit sings" at Maplewood several times a month. Hayes's daughter Jennie has asked Susan to say something at the service and, along with Scotty, to sing. It's not all that surprising to see Brooke and Susan here, given the close ties Hayes's daughter and the family have maintained with the facility for more than two years. Also, because Brooke and Susan, unlike most Maplewood employees, are not on the clock, they can take time away from work to come out in the middle of a workday.

What's astonishing is that seven RAs are here, women who have no "sick days" or "vacation days" or "personal days" they can take. Perks like these are nonexistent at Maplewood, or industry-wide, for bottom-of-the-rung caregivers. Three RAs are here on their day off. Spending part of it at the funeral, offering this day to the memory of Hayes, is a truly magnanimous gift.

Two others will have to leave early to clock in for swing. The other two are supposed to be on duty right now. They have scrounged to find people to trade shifts with them, favors they will have to repay at times when they may not want to repay them. These are all women who don't have the luxury of time: Inez with her husband in a wheelchair; Jasmine and her seven-year-old whom she rarely sees; Heidi, who takes care of an ailing grandmother when she's not taking care of her Maplewood residents; Cathy with a home life so ugly and chaotic that you don't want to know the details. I think of all the people who don't know about the world of eldercare but think they do, people who have read the occasional sensational news story about abuse and neglect and think institutional caregivers are at best insensitive and coldhearted and at worst perverts and criminals. I wish they could see these women who have come to Hayes's funeral.

The service begins with Susan at the microphone talking about how important music was to Hayes at "this time in his life." She has to say "this time in his life" and not "when he lived at Maplewood" or "his last years with Alzheimer's" because Jennie has requested there be no references like this. It's odd, given that at least the immediate family seemed to make peace with Hayes's illness, but I do understand. They would all rather remember their father or grandfather as the man I see in the color photograph in the pamphlet the family has created for the service. This Hayes is thirty or forty pounds heavier than the one I knew, yet he is still trim. He stands straight and tall, dressed in a red flannel shirt and brown checked slacks. (He dressed better at Maplewood, I must say.) His face is square and strong jawed, the resolute face of a hardworking Swede, a stern face, not impish like the one I remember. He looks vital and healthy, outdoorsy, untroubled, invincible.

Later, when I get home, I study a photograph of my mother that I keep on the bookshelf in my writing room. It must be from the late 1980s. My mother and my aunt are flanking their mother, who was then in her early nineties and a real pistol. Nanny, as I called my maternal grandmother, looks as if the camera caught her in mid-laugh. My mother is smiling too, her long oval face flushed and alive. I study the face in the photograph, looking for hints of the woman she would become just a few years later. I can't see it, and I'm glad.

Susan, standing alongside the pulpit, is talking about Hayes's love of music. She manages not to cry—but just barely. This is a huge accomplishment for Susan, a woman who chokes up three or four times during the course of any given day. The expression "wearing your heart on your sleeve" was made for Susan. I'm glad she holds it together because somehow it feels like we who are not his family, we who knew him only in the very last part of his long life, do not have the right to cry. Still, when the pianist begins to play "You are my sunshine," and everyone in the chapel sings, in amazing impromptu harmony, the tears start streaming down my cheeks. Next to me, Inez is sobbing.

The minister comes to the pulpit. He's mid-fiftyish, with a trim beard, and he is wearing clogs (true to the "I went to divinity school in the sixties" stereotype, his guitar is leaning against the wall). The sermon, which is a good one, is about acceptance, the power of acceptance, how this is, if you are a believer, a gift from God. Acceptance is a kind of grace, the minister says. You don't work for it. You don't earn it. It just is. Hayes, he says, was a man who accepted. I am thinking that the minister means Hayes accepted his fate, his disease, and, at least in his daughter's eyes, became a better man for it. But the minister is talking about Hayes's unconditional acceptance of others. When you were in his presence, you felt accepted, the minister says. This is such a simple statement, so humble and understated. The minister does not go on with the usual platitudes about how loving or giving or selfless Hayes was, about the meaning of his life, about his place in the family or in the community. He talks only about how Hayes made each person feel accepted. That's what the minister says he kept hearing from Hayes's children and grandchildren when he talked to them. This gift Hayes gave is perhaps deeper and more important than the gift of love. It speaks to openheartedness and open-mindedness. It speaks to forgiveness. It speaks a language I barely know. This is not a gift I ever received from my mother, nor one I gave her.

A microphone is set up just below the pulpit. The minister asks who would like to say a few words about Hayes. Jennie, the dutiful daughter, reads a poem Hayes wrote in her autograph book when she was ten. Another daughter tells a funny story about how Hayes, who learned to fly in the 1950s, sometimes awoke the family at dawn by buzzing the house with his little Cessna. A son who looks exactly like the Hayes in the color photograph, reads a Wendell Berry poem. Then another daughter, then four grandchildren, each with little stories about Hayes taking the time to be with them, hiking, fishing, flying kites. It all sounds sincere, not like those eulogies where you know the eulogizer has carefully edited history or is biting his or her tongue, where everyone knows there's a subtext, those untold stories, those dark moments. Of course, there are untold stories and dark moments—what family does not have these? Hayes was no saint. But it seems he was a truly good man, a hardworking man of few words who lived a quiet, dignified, hardworking life.

Cathy from Maplewood comes to the microphone. Her voice is shaking, a combination of emotion and nerves. She's never spoken in front of a crowd before. "No matter how bad it was for me at home," she says—and looking at her, just looking at her, the hard face, the bad skin, the missing teeth, you can see how hard it is for her at home, how hard her whole life has been—"no matter how hard," she says, "when I went to work I felt so much love from Hayes and Mabel." This sounds so formulaic that it almost doesn't ring true. But I know it is true. I know that Cathy, despite that she makes minimum wage at a job that carries negative status, is in fact nourished by the work. She gets something back. She is loved and appreciated at work.

The lady at the piano plays "I'm forever blowing bubbles," a really silly song Hayes loved to sing, and before she gets to the end of the first line, there are bubbles everywhere, iridescent bubbles floating in the air, floating up in front of the stained-glass windows, up to the wooden rafters, courtesy of every kid in the chapel under the age of ten. Hayes's family has planned this, has put out the word for all kids to come to church with those forty-nine-cent containers of soap bubble solution with the plastic wands inside. Now they are waving the wands back and forth leaving trails of bubbles, giggling. Their parents aren't shushing them. Their parents, we all, are singing loudly, with abandon, following the words on the song sheets handed out at the beginning of the service. The pianist segues into "It's a long way to Tipperary," a popular World War I–era song that Hayes would have heard as a kid.

Susan and Scotty sing the last song of the afternoon, "Amazing Grace," a beautiful song, sad and hopeful at the same time. I know it's about God and redemption, and I know I'm only a tentative believer, but the song always gets to me. I wish I could sing along, but the key is too high. When the song ends, the minister surveys the entire chapel-in-the-round, slowly swiveling his head and turning his body, taking us all in, making eye contact, or so it seems to me. The room is silent, waiting. If Hayes's spirit is here, I feel as if it's waiting too. I think I see the minister taking a long, deep breath. He looks down for a moment. Then he takes a step away from the pulpit. "Go in peace," he says. He means us, but I think he also means Hayes.

In the Fellowship Hall, where the family is hosting a reception, there are four tables of Hayes memorabilia—a photo of his mother holding baby Hayes in 1912; Hayes in knee pants squinting into the sun on the farm in Alberta; Hayes one of seventeen seniors posing for his high school graduation picture in 1931; Hayes sitting on the sideboard of an old Ford flatbed truck loaded with Christmas trees bound for Los Angeles; Hayes perched atop a tractor; Hayes in his machine shop. There are plaques and certificates, a wartime commendation, business cards, a pilot's log. Along the opposite wall, there are three tables crowded with thirty-seven plates of cookies, confections, brownies, bars, and fudge, and not a single store-bought item among them.

19

I take a week off after the funerals. I need time to accept that Rose and Hayes are both gone. When you work with the sick elderly, you know their days are numbered, but knowing that they will die and the *fact* of them dying are two different things. I am very slowly learning not to be unnerved by what is really, when I think about it, just the rhythm of life. In our culture, it's easy to shield yourself from that rhythm, to not hear it or feel it, to think you exist outside it. Your world is healthy and forever young. Death happens elsewhere, to invisible, anonymous people. But here at Maplewood, I am unshielded.

I've heard it said that when a person has an illness like Alzheimer's, death is "a blessing," or that so-and-so "wouldn't have wanted to live this way." This, I guess, is supposed to be solace for the grieving family, but I find the remarks disquieting. They deny the person's humanity, as if the person ceased to be entitled to life because he or she had a disease. They sever life from death, health from illness, as if all these events were not a natural and inevitable part of the human experience. Philosophy aside, I find it hard to think of *these* two deaths as "blessings." I see Hayes with the filtered sun on his handsome face tapping his toy drum in time to a Glenn Miller tune. I see Rose licking the chocolate from her lips after eating a cookie.

Maybe some people think these small, momentary pleasures are too little to live for. They remember Dad or Grandpa when he used to go fishing. They remember Mom or Grandma hosting holiday dinners. Then comes Alzheimer's, and Grandpa or Grandma, Mom or Dad can no longer live the life they lived before. Things change. *Everything changes.* Their lives, their families' lives, are transformed. Is the new life, the post-disease life, not worth living? Is death what a person with Alzheimer's would long for if he or she had a lucid moment?

I don't know. I used to think I knew when it was my own mother. I used to think anything was better than her life with Alzheimer's, even death. But I am questioning that belief now. I see that it came from fear and aversion, from the fact that I didn't try to understand her new life. I didn't even see it. And I never knew the person she was with Alzheimer's. For me, she was a disease, not a person. But I knew Hayes. I knew Rose. I knew them only as they were after the disease changed them. And I saw something there. I saw value in their much-diminished selves. And so the double deaths—the "passings" as we say at Maplewood—hit me hard.

When I finally come back to work, I feel as if I've forgotten everything I ever knew. I struggle with the chores. I struggle to get everyone fed, forgetting the details of diets, forgetting who drinks coffee, who likes juice, who can't eat fish. I try and fail to find the rhythm of the workday. Where is that zone I thought I was in? Where is that good little worker who earned a star? What happened to that transformation I thought I went through when I danced with Rose? Maplewood feels disconcertingly peaceful without Rose wandering the hallways. The neighborhood is unnervingly quiet without Hayes yelling, *I'm itchy, I'm itchy. Rub my back.* I have come back to an off-kilter universe.

Another change, a big one, is that I've decided to work swing shift, 2:30 in the afternoon to 10:30 at night. Now that it's autumn, I need to be home in the morning to help get the kids fed and ready and off to school. But changing my schedule is more than a matter of family responsibilities. I've decided that I want to experience another part of the day with the residents. On swing, I will not be waking them up but rather putting them to sleep. I will be serving one meal, not two, which some RAs say makes the shift more relaxed. It's not as hectic in the neighborhoods on swing because the majority of the planned activities—sing-alongs, visits by animals, exercise classes—are scheduled for mornings. Also, by 6:00 p.m. the administrative staff has left the building, which, I am told, changes the workplace ambience—for the better, say my coworkers.

I've been looking forward to working the new shift, so it comes as an unhappy surprise that my first days back at work after the funeral seem both long and unpleasant. At first I think this is the emotional fallout from the two deaths complicated by my difficulty adjusting to the new hours. I am actually getting considerably less sleep on swing shift than on day shift. I no longer have to wake up at 5:00 a.m., but I can't sleep all that late because of the kids' school schedule. When I get off work at 10:30, I am tired but wired. I need to decompress for at least several hours, so I'm rarely in bed before two—and then up to start the day five hours later. I wonder how other swing-shift RAs with kids handle this, the ones who don't have supportive husbands shouldering part of the load like I do, the ones who don't have happy, stable, well-adjusted kids, the ones who can't count on their car starting every morning.

But there's something else going on, some bigger reason that the job all of a sudden feels so much harder. There is, I am discovering, a special rhythm to an Alzheimer's day. In the late afternoon, just a few hours in to my shift, and through the evening, some of my residents go through a transformation. Their behavior changes dramatically and so does, as a consequence, the dynamic of the neighborhood and the job I do.

One night it's Marianne who loses it. Because she has created this alternative reality for herself—either as an administrator at Maplewood or, sometimes, a retired exec here for R&R—she mostly protects herself from the confusion and dislocation she might normally experience. Or at least that's what I thought when I was part of Marianne's morning and early afternoon life. But at night, at least this night, something is different. Marianne generally keeps to herself, showing up for meals impeccably dressed and carrying her Coach purse. She has been known to obsess about phone calls she thinks she's getting or luncheon engagements she thinks she has, and one time she did give the Med Aide a hard time about taking a new pill, but in general Marianne is prim and proper, self-contained, mannerly, and polite. Only tonight she is not. Tonight she is pacing the neighborhood, clearly angry. She sits for a moment at the dining room table and empties out her purse on a placemat.

"It was in here this morning. I know it was here," she says, her voice rising. She gets up, stalks over to her room, and begins to open drawers.

"What are you looking for?" I ask. I keep my voice pleasant and conversational, thinking this might ground her. She looks up at me, disgusted.

"You know," she says. "You probably took them."

"Took what?"

"My keys, my goddamned car keys. I need my car keys." I'm

stymied about what to do. With Marianne I've almost always practiced "validation therapy," buying into whatever fantasy she was living, rarely questioning whatever her take on reality was at the moment. But I can't do that in this situation. I decide to be honest.

"Marianne," I say, "you don't have a car anymore. You sold it when you came here." She shakes her head.

"That's ridiculous," she says. "I just drove the car yesterday. It's out in the parking lot. Now give me my keys." I try to reason with her, which only makes her angrier. I try to "redirect," which makes her angrier still. The drama is escalating. I've got to do something. I've got to get myself out of the equation because now she's even madder at me than she is about the missing keys.

I call Susan on the walkie. It's almost 6:00 p.m., but thankfully she's still in the building. Susan sits and listens quietly to what Marianne has to say. I get out of the way. When I circle back a few minutes later and eavesdrop from the threshold of her room, I hear that they are having a calm conversation. Susan is patting Marianne's arm and telling her how smart she was to get rid of that old car.

The next night it's Eloise's turn to howl. Eloise is moody even during the day, so I am not surprised when she walks up to me after dinner, grabs my hand, and says, "I'm so stupid. How could someone be so stupid?" I don't know exactly what she's referring to, and it doesn't really matter. I give her the usual assurances, but she is not buying any of it. "I'm so stupid. How can you stand to be around someone as stupid as me?" I tell her I love being around her. I tell her she is important to me. But clearly, I am not getting through to her. Whatever mental place she's in, she's stuck there. I reassure her a dozen, two dozen times that she is not stupid, that everything is okay. She follows me around for most of the next two and a half hours, berating herself, inconsolable. Finally, blessedly, at 8:30 she tires herself out, and I am able to put her to bed.

Then, two nights later, it's Addie. I am kneeling next to her wheelchair telling her it's bedtime. She looks down at me with a hard stare. "I want to go home," she yells.

"You are home, Addie," I say gently. Then, quickly changing the subject: "Did you see Stan today?" Stan is her son who visits just about every afternoon. He is a calm, steady fellow with a gentle sense of humor who, it is immediately clear to me, visits his mother out of love, not obligation. Watching him lean in to quietly talk to her, seeing how tenderly he holds her hand, is the best thing about swing shift.

"I want to go home, and I'M GOING HOME RIGHT NOW!" She is screaming.

"Okay, Addie, okay."

"Do you want to go to hell?" she yells at me. "Well, then just stop this shitting stuff." I guess she means stop bullshitting her. I'm kneeling in front of her, my hand resting on her arm trying to figure out what to do next, when she grabs my ponytail. She yanks it hard.

"I'm gonna kill you," she yells. "I'm gonna kill someone." She is fierce and wild-eyed, hyperventilating. I'm not frightened for my safety. Addie is wheelchair-bound. She can't hurt anyone. But I am afraid for her. She is in distress, and I don't know how to help. I keep my voice calm. I reassure her. But, like Eloise a few days ago, she's not having any of it. *No one loves me. I'm going to kill you. I hate you. You are trying to hurt me. You are abusing me.* Yes, she uses the word *abusing*, and I wonder why this word remains as part of her limited vocabulary.

I say, Addie, look at me. I am here to help you. I would never hurt you. I wheel her into her bedroom, find her nightgown, and start to undress her. She rears up in her chair. "You're a liar. You're a liar," she screams at me. She keeps this up as I toilet her, hand her a toothbrush, guide her hand, wash her face, transfer her from wheelchair to bed—no mean feat, as she outweighs me—surround her with pillows, tuck her in. All the while I am keeping up a litany of *No one is going to hurt you . . . you are safe here,* and she is keeping up a litany of *I'm going to kill you.* Neither of us is listening to the other. I get her in bed. I close the bedroom door behind me and stand weeping in the hallway.

I've read about this phenomenon. The literature calls it "sundowning" or "sundowner's syndrome." But I had understood it as a problem related to mixing up night and day, something about people with Alzheimer's wandering or getting restless late in the day. It sounded pretty harmless. Places like Maplewood, the new generation of Alzheimer's care facilities, acknowledge and understand restlessness and wandering as an issue, and they are designed to deal with it. The architecture here facilitates wandering, with broad hallways and unlocked doors leading to protected courtyards. Not having to constrain or limit people when they become restless means fewer "behaviors."

But the restlessness is only part of it. There is also agitation, confusion, depression, delusions. A psychiatric text calls the phenomenon "recurrent nocturnal delirium." In other words, normally complacent or well-mannered or quiet folks can go nuts when the sun goes down. One theory is that frustrations and sensory stimulation build up throughout the day so that by day's end a person is ready to blow. The world, even the controlled world within the walls of a place like Maplewood, can be a confusing, anxiety-producing environment for a person with Alzheimer's. To someone with severely impaired short-term memory everything can seem new, each trip to the bathroom a journey to a foreign land, each visitor a stranger. How much newness can one person take? How many times during the day can a person handle being baffled?

Not to conflate the beginning of life with the end, but babies confront similar challenges to those faced by people with Alzheimer's. Thrust into a world they do not understand, surrounded by strangers who make noises they can't comprehend, awash in alien sights and smells, babies have a lot to handle. The world must seem to them much like the world appears to a person with Alzheimer's. Not surprisingly, like sundowners, babies are known to fall apart at the end of the day—or right before nap time. But babies have a built-in escape valve: they sleep, often eighteen hours a day, able to retreat from the confusion of all these new stimuli.

And, of course, babies learn. They decode the environment, the language, facial expressions, smells, tastes, textures, item by item, piece by piece, every day. And so their world, unlike the Alzheimer's world, becomes progressively less strange, increasingly comfortable and easier to navigate. I bet it also makes a difference, maybe a huge difference, that babies, unlike the elderly, are constantly hugged and held and stroked and smiled at. We do a lot of touching at Maplewood. Susan believes every person needs to be hugged every day and that some of our residents may not have felt the comfort of human touch for years. Still, the pat on the shoulder or squeeze on the arm or peck on the cheek cannot compare to the enveloping, nurturing world many infants are lucky enough to experience.

This theory of sundowning, the idea that a long day lived in a consistently confusing environment might lead to "nocturnal delirium," makes sense to me. It seems almost obvious. In fact, the more I think about it, the more I marvel that only *some* people with Alzheimer's are sundowners. But this isn't the only theory. Apparently there's also the thought that sundowning might be akin to SAD—seasonal affective disorder—the depression and lethargy some people experience in winter when there is less light. This is a biochemical explanation having to do with the pineal gland and its secretion of melatonin, a hormone that, among other things, regulates sleep-wake cycles. I start to read about all this, to background myself on the issue as I encounter it in the neighborhood, but the purely scientific explanation doesn't do much for me. It feels divorced from the reality of my residents' lives. At any rate, all this reading is not making swing shift any easier.

For the first time in many weeks, Jasmine and I again find ourselves working the same shift on the same day. She's across the courtyard in neighborhood 4, home to Caroline, the former Radio City Music Hall Rockette, and Jeanette, the woman for whom every day is the day she's going to pack to go home. I see Jasmine briefly after dinner when I take a detour and roll my meal cart through her neighborhood on the way to the kitchen. She looks wonderful. Her skin is glowing, her eyes are bright. She is smiling. I want to know what's going on, but I'll have to wait until lights out. If both of us can get all our residents down early, we might have a few minutes to talk.

Miraculously, it works out that way. By 8:45 everyone's in bed, and we have a few minutes before we must start in on our end-of-shift chores. It's a lovely fall evening, cool but not cold, a sky full of stars. Jasmine is already out in the courtyard between our two neighborhoods, sitting on one of the plastic patio chairs smoking when I can finally take a break. The first thing she tells me, before I even sit down, is that she gave notice today.

"So that's why you look so happy," I say. She laughs. We've both just hit the three-month employment mark, which, according to what we've heard from our coworkers and the administrators, is about the average life span of an RA here. A significant subset of people quit after their three-day training period; most quit after three months. And then there are the occasional living saints like Calm Guam Frances who are in it for the long haul. Even taking into account the often chaotic private lives of people who work jobs like this, lives full of upheaval that can cause frequent job changes (losing an apartment, getting a car repossessed), burnout, by itself, is a major issue. Jasmine, who has been taking extra shifts whenever she can, even occasionally working back-to-back shifts, while juggling life as a single mother and, by the way, battling clinical depression, is, she says, officially burned out.

"Can you imagine doing this full time?" she says, lighting a second cigarette from the butt of the first.

"*You* did it full-time," I say. "You even did it overtime."

"No, I mean *really* full-time, as in twenty-four hours a day, as in this guy is my husband, and I take care of him 24/7."

I've thought about this many times since I started working here. Family members who come to visit, especially the daughters, have sought me out to say how bad they feel that they could no longer care for Mom at home. They bring her to Maplewood after they have exhausted themselves as caregivers, after months of sleepless nights, after three back-to-back shifts a day, every day. They seem ashamed, like it is a crime, or at least a dereliction of duty, to place Mom in a residential facility. I think about my father's life when he was caring for my mother at home, alone, with no help, no adult day care, no respite. If it takes us—the single-shift "professional" caregivers—three months to burn out, I consider it a genuine miracle that family members last as long as they do. I also think—and I've told wives and daughters and sons this—that, at a certain point, an Alzheimer's facility, a decent one like Maplewood, is the best, most humane, most loving place their mom can be.

I will be sorry to see Jasmine go. Although we haven't been able to spend much time together, our three intense days of training plus dozens of conversations on the fly have bonded us. With her departure, I will be the only one remaining of the five who went through orientation back in July.

"So what's the plan?" I ask. "Whatever it is, you look happy about it." Jasmine tells me her sister is moving up from California and that they've found a small apartment in a nearby city. Jasmine has saved enough money to enroll part-time at a community college. She'll need to work part-time, she tells me, but her son won't have to be in twelve-hour-a-day day care because her sister can take care of him when *she's* not working. The two of them have negotiated what sounds like a complicated but doable work-school-home schedule. Jasmine is excited to be moving on. I tell her how proud I am of her. She's really taking control of her life.

"And, oh yeah, I didn't tell you the best part," she says, and goes on to talk about Willie, this guy she and her sister met at Target while shopping for kitchen stuff. "He is sooo cute. And such a *bad* boy." Jasmine is twenty-four, looks thirty, has lived enough to be forty, but right now sounds fourteen. I want to say, *Jasmine, listen to yourself. . . . Wasn't it a bad boy you fell for at sixteen who got you pregnant and left? Aren't you through with bad boys?* Meanwhile, she's smiling and smoking and telling me that Willie has curly black hair and a smooth chest and a wicked smile—and, incidentally, has been out of work for six months.

I drive home in a daze. It's after 11:00 p.m. when I park the car in the garage. In the house, all the lights are out except for the one in the master bedroom. The kids are asleep. My husband is probably reading in bed. I walk into the kitchen, not bothering to turn on the light, and make a beeline for the refrigerator. I stand there, in front of the open door, illuminated by the 40-watt bulb, and eat my way through the top two shelves—cottage cheese, yogurt, bean dip, olives, it doesn't matter. Then I go upstairs and tell my husband that I'm quitting the job.

20

My mother had been in Oregon living at the care facility for five months when my father started making noises about bringing her back home to New York. Having her out here had not been a great success. She was losing ground—ground she undoubtedly would have lost wherever she was—but she wasn't "wherever." She was with me. And although I understood that I had no control over the progress of her disease, that didn't keep me from feeling responsible. My father—Mr. I'm-in-Charge-and-You're-Not—had relinquished the reins and entrusted me with her care. This was my watch, and I held myself accountable for anything that happened on it. Her time with me was also my chance to show what a good daughter I was.

In this little fantasy I had plotted many months before, I would rescue both my father, who was exhausted from round-the-clock caregiving, and my mother, who needed better care than my father could give. He would get eight hours of sleep a night. He would be able to play tennis with his pals and eat out at Kwan Ming, his favorite Chinese restaurant. Meanwhile, in residential care, my mother would be dressed every day in clean clothes and sleep between clean sheets. She would eat three meals of wholesome food. She would get regular showers and be toileted every two hours.

But the fantasy was not just about how my intervention would significantly improve both their lives, it was also—and maybe just as much—about what I would get out of the whole deal. My father would have to grudgingly admit that I was worthy of respect. My mother, although lost in the haze of her disease, would sense my filial devotion and maybe see it as love, and maybe love me back. In this heartwarming Hallmark movie, I was the generous, healing center of my fragmented family, the estranged daughter who made everything right at the end.

Only it hadn't worked out that way. As the weeks, and then months, went by, although I visited my mother dutifully, we had had few moments of connection, and those were fleeting. Mostly she got thinner and frailer, less articulate, more repetitive, less agreeable, more distant. After a while, she was too far gone to sit for the hairdresser who came to her facility every Thursday, so her once well coiffed head of soft, wavy dyed-copper hair went back to iron gray, alternately springy and frizzy depending on the humidity. All her muscles were tight and tense—she might have had Parkinson's, according to the doctor—including her jaw muscles. It was almost impossible to get her to open her mouth wide enough to get a toothbrush in. Her breath stank. If she went back to New York, what would my father say when he saw her? If she went back to New York, I lost all hope of being the family heroine.

When he asked for her return, I wasn't sure why he wanted her back. My first thought was that he could no longer deal with having someone else, especially me, in charge. My next thought was that he wanted to save money. The Oregon facility had raised its rates and was, my father thought (correctly), nickel-and-diming him, charging him for items he had thought were included in the monthly fee. He was always getting separate little bills, and he hated that. It was only much later that it occurred to me that he might have wanted her back because, after forty-eight years of marriage, he needed to be part of her daily life. He needed to be part of the end game.

But I didn't see that then. At the time, I battled him for control of my mother's future. He went out looking for facilities on Long Island, told me about them, and I found something wrong with each one: the caregiver-resident ratio was too high, the facility had no activity director, the available room was on the second floor. She was settled in out here, I told him. Disrupting her routine would cause anxiety and confusion. I used every argument I could think of. Going head-to-head with my father was, I had learned through years of doing just that, a kamikaze mission. Still I did it.

He found a place just fifteen minutes away from his house, the suburban split-level I had grown up in. He liked this facility. The grounds were pretty. The director was smart. The price was right. I argued that it was not a dedicated Alzheimer's facility, that she wouldn't get the level of care she got out here. We spent weeks sparring on the phone, but he was unbudgeable.

I hired the same geriatric nurse who had accompanied her on the westbound flight six months before to take care of her on the return flight. On the morning of departure, I went out to the facility one last time to pick her up. One of the caregivers had somehow managed to give her a home perm. The staff, I'm sure, thought this was a good thing, but the results were ghastly. My mother looked like she was wearing a wig made of steel wool pads. I hardly recognized her. On the drive out to the airport, I told her where we were going and what would be happening.

In a few hours you'll be seeing Dad again, I said. I don't know if she understood, but she didn't respond. I filled the silence with chatter, talking nonstop during the thirty-minute drive to the airport.

In the photograph I asked the nurse to take right before the two of them boarded the plane, my mother and I stand in such obvious contrast that the picture, when I studied it later, appeared to be a set-up, the work of an exceptionally heavy handed visual artist trying to make a point about life and death: My mother pasty-faced, vacant-eyed, shrunken, a head of steel wool, a smear of orangey-red lipstick; me looking Amazonian, towering over her, my posture too erect, my face too alive, my color too good, as if I were hogging all the life force. I stared at the photo for days, showed it to no one, then tore it up.

Despite declarations to the contrary, I have yet to quit my job at Maplewood. That's not because I've changed my mind about quitting but because my other life has conveniently intervened to give me a long break. Although I never forget my privileged position as I work at the facility—a position that allows me, un-like my coworkers, to work when I want to, change shifts when I want to, and stay in the same neighborhood—I sometimes do forget, or at least don't think about, the existence of my non-Maplewood working life. But in fact I do have another life, and it happens that my publisher wants me to do some bookstore readings. Two events are scheduled for Seattle and neatly coin-cide with the start of my oldest son's first term at the University of Washington. I call Christine, who coordinates the RAs' work schedules, and tell her not to put me down for any shifts for the next pay period. "You're coming back, aren't you?" she asks. I give her an elaborate nonanswer.

My son and I prepare for his departure by spending days

cloistered in his upstairs bedroom listening to Tom Petty and culling through stacks of old term papers, English essays, lab notes, Boy Scout badge books, and Harry Potter hardbacks, clearing shelves of broken model rockets, engineering club experiments, and Disney souvenirs. We pack boxes of electronics, duffel bags of clean clothes, special twin X-long sheets for his dorm bed, a small, cheap microwave oven, three pounds of red licorice.

In Seattle, we have several days together before his dorm opens. We stay at a nice hotel and eat out at a different Thai restaurant every night. He accompanies me to the reading events. We explore the city. We rent bikes and follow the Burke Gilman Trail north along the shore of Lake Washington. In the room at night we order up a "game cart" and sprawl on our separate queen beds asking each other Trivial Pursuit questions for hours. We don't keep score. We play Monopoly and cheat. We play blackjack for jelly beans. Then, early in the morning of our fourth day together, I drive him to his dorm, help him set up the room, put away his clothes, make his bed, tack up the posters, and then hang out until, as hard as I try, I can't think of one more reason to stay.

For him, this is the beginning of a grand adventure. I know that. I remember how free and light I felt the afternoon my father said good-bye to me in the lobby of Allison Hall, my freshman dorm at Northwestern. I was launched into the rest of my life, fearless and clueless as only an eighteen-year-old can be. Now I'm on the other side of the equation: the parent waving good-bye, the one left on the launch pad. What is the beginning of an era for my son is the end of one for me. And it is an era I am not yet ready to let go of. I know so many people who talk about how glad they are to finally get their teenagers out of the house. Not me.

I've spent the last eighteen years helping to create a happy, functional family that does the things the family I was born into never did—like talk to each other, like enjoy each other's quirkiness, like laugh together at the dining room table. Now I am saying good-bye to one-fifth of that family. I know my son will be home for vacations. I know he'll come home for at least the first summer. But we will never be the same family again. I know that he must look forward, not back, and that I must not do anything to obscure his vision or impede his journey. I can't tell him how torn up I feel. I can't tell him how I wish I could stop the clock. I do tell my husband, but he is far less emotional about this moment than I am. He tells me how important it is for a young man to leave home. I tell my friends, and they advise me to convert my son's bedroom to an in-home gym. Four days after saying good-bye, it is still impossible for me to talk about my son without feeling my throat close up. I don't know what to do with myself.

So I go back to work.

I go back selfish and needy. I go back hungry for the emotional sustenance I get at Maplewood. It's odd. This is the most draining work I've ever done, but as I am drained, I am also filled, and I think the equation often works in my favor. Right now, I need to have these folks in neighborhood 3 need me, the way my son once needed me. Since I left him at the dorm, I've been reliving those times during the past eighteen years that I've been able to soothe him, to banish pain or fear or hurt with those magical powers a parent has, a mother has. But the magic doesn't last. Life gets more complicated. Kids get smart. They understand soon enough that you are not really all-powerful, that you can't make everything right with a long hug or a cup of hot chocolate. But for a time, for a moment, you have that power, and it is the best feeling in the world: the ability to bring peace to another human being, to heal all manner of hurts. And that's a good part of what I do, just about every day in neighborhood 3. The magic comes in the midst of exhausting physical labor, of the unpleasant, intimate work of caring for aging human bodies and of the grinding, exasperating, petty annoyances of a minimum-wage job. But the magic does come. And today, I need to feel it.

When I walk into the neighborhood, there is Eloise sitting at the dining room table dressed in her navy blue sweater drinking her usual cup of lukewarm decaf. I may have come back to work to be needed, but the very first thing I do is seek succor, not give it. It doesn't matter than Eloise has Alzheimer's, that she does not remember my name or the conversations we've had. Today, this afternoon, now, I need Eloise. I don't stop to debrief the day-shift RA. I don't stop to check the comm log. I don't stop to put my lunch in the little refrigerator. I go immediately to Eloise and tell her about taking my son to college. As I start to talk, I start to weep. She takes my hand and listens intently. I see how hard she is working to follow my sentences, to track my thoughts.

"And how often has he been in this situation?" she asks, when I stop talking long enough to look for a Kleenex. So, she hasn't followed what I've been saying. I feel defeated, deflated, and silly. What do I expect from this woman who is so deep into dementia that she cannot dress herself, that she sometimes does not remember which room is hers? I have to answer her, although I'm not quite sure what she is asking.

"He just started college," I say. "I just left him at school last week." She nods. I get up from the chair I have pulled next to hers and begin to walk away. I have to start working. I have to read the comm log and catch up on the service plans. I have two showers to give. Eloise grabs hold of my arm as I take a step away.

"You can't hold on to them forever," she says. "Everything can't stay the same." Wisdom, it seems, exists outside of memory.

At dinner, Addie has a series of little anxiety attacks. I comfort her, speaking in long, rambling, soporific sentences. I tell her, again and again, that it's just another meal, just another evening, the same people gathered around the same table. My voice is low and a little singsong. It's a voice I suddenly recognize. I talked to my oldest son like this. He was eight. We were saying good-bye to him in the parking lot of Camp Meriwether. It would be his first-ever week away from home. I talked to my second son like this. He was seven and had broken his arm falling from the tree house. I held him on my lap at the hospital while they took X-rays. I talked to my daughter like this. She was six. She had run over to the sidelines in tears after having kicked the soccer ball in the wrong direction, past her own team's goalie and into the net. It is a mother's voice. It calms and soothes. It helps the moment pass.

That night, I take my time putting the residents to bed, the ones who need my complete attention, Old Frances and Addie, the new guy Larry, Eloise. The chores are the same: I toilet them, change them into nightclothes, brush their teeth. But when I finally get them in bed, each in turn, I take a long moment before I go on to the next. I sit on the side of Old Frances's bed and stroke her soft, almost unlined cheek. I lay my head next to Addie's on the pillow. I pat Larry's arm as his eyelids flutter shut. I sit in Eloise's room, in the chair by her bed, and listen as her breathing slows and deepens.

This, my first time back in two weeks, is coincidentally Jasmine's last day on the job. I didn't know I would get to see her again. After final chores, we meet in the outside courtyard between our two neighborhoods. It's early October and getting cold now. I ask Jasmine if her sister has arrived yet, if her apartment is ready to move in, what classes she's planning to take at the junior college in January. I stay away from the subject of Willie, the bad boy. If they are still seeing each other, I don't want to hear about it. If she's crazy in love, I don't want to know.

I tell Jasmine about driving my son up to Seattle to start school, about how hard this transition is for me, how I wish I could go back a few weeks, a few months, a few years and stop time. I want to live in that moment when all three kids are at home, and we go out to the movies on rainy Saturday afternoons, eat pizza on the living room floor and call it a picnic, make overly elaborate doomed sand fortresses at the beach, take day hikes in the woods with "energy pills" (M&M's) in our pockets.

Jasmine smokes and listens. I go on for too long. She lights another cigarette. "There's never been a time I wanted to stay frozen in," she says. "Things have just never been that good." If she wasn't so matter-of-fact about it, I'd feel terrible for going on and on about what sounds in the retelling like a perfect little life. She gives me a big smile, wide enough so I can see all her missing molars. "I hope some day I feel about my life the way you feel about yours," she says.

21

I've mostly thought about how everything here changes all the time, residents dying and new ones arriving, RAs quitting and new ones hiring on, and lately, people you know becoming people you don't know when the sun goes down. But it also seems, at the same time, that nothing changes at all, that all of us—residents and families, workers and administrators—live in this permanent, immutable *now*. It must be the *nowness* of this disease that, in stealing the past and obscuring the future, forces us, the healthy and the ill, to stay in the moment. There is a rhythm to Maplewood days, quick and hurried on the surface as we RAs rush from chore to chore, but plodding and deliberate underneath as the residents live their slow-motion lives. The counterpoint is almost hypnotic.

Maybe this is what brings me back. The place has hypnotized me. Maplewood pulls at me, metal filings to a magnet. The residents draw me close. The challenge of meeting their needs is as powerful a lure as the feeling of being needed. And so, despite my decision to quit, I'm back on the October schedule, back to putting on my khaki pants (tighter now than they once were—Calm Guam Frances was right: against all logic, you gain weight working here), back to wearing my ugly polyester shirt and my half-apron stuffed with latex gloves, back on swing.

I am not, however, back in the zone. At least not yet. Although the routines and rhythms of the place are so familiar as to be imprinted on my brain by now, I can't go on auto-pilot here, I can't just fit myself back into a niche. New residents bring significant new challenges.

Larry isn't exactly new—he arrived several weeks ago—but because I've been gone much of that time I have maybe two days worth of experience caring for him. He is undemanding—quiet, docile, even-tempered—but he needs a lot of help, as much as or more than anyone else in the neighborhood. The kicker is that Larry is a big man, a full-sized, broad-shouldered six-footer. Helping him into and out of bed, into and out of chairs is no small task. It takes not just energy, strength, and stamina but strategy and advance planning. It's not like helping Old Frances, who is so small and light that, in a pinch, I can pick her up and carry her. I have to learn how much I can depend on my own muscles and how much Larry can do. I have to learn what he understands, what he likes, what he can tolerate.

The afternoon trudges on filled with the usual litany of chores, my job made more difficult by Larry's inability to do anything without help. After dinner, during which Larry manages to wear more of his meal than he eats—I am just too busy with the others to sit and hand feed him—I wheel him into the living room so he won't be alone. When I pass by a few minutes later, I know he needs my help by the look in his eyes. He is sitting in his wheelchair watching the Katharine Hepburn–Spencer Tracy movie I've put in the VCR. But there's Addie to deal with first, then Old Frances. In between, I stop by Larry's wheelchair, pat him on the shoulder, and tell him I'll be with him as soon as I can. I sprint to Pam's room, then back again. Finally, I am kneeling down beside Larry's wheelchair. The sweatshirt I put on him a half hour ago has a trail of applesauce down the front to which assorted biscuit crumbs have adhered. His big gnarled hands are shaking a little. He tells me he has to go to the bathroom.

"I'm so sorry you had to wait," I say as I unlock the wheelchair brakes and move him toward his room.

"I guess that's my job now," he says. "To wait."

I think about Larry's comment for the rest of the day. I think about the time old people spend waiting, not just in places like Maplewood but throughout the eldercare system—nursing homes, assisted living, rehab, any facility that houses those who are no longer able to take care of themselves. They lie in bed, wide awake at 5:00 a.m., waiting for a caregiver to help them get up and dressed. They sit at the table waiting for meals, the first ones wheeled in fifteen or twenty minutes early because it takes so much time to get everyone in their places. They wait, like Larry, to be taken to the bathroom. They wait for attention.

The problem is understaffing. The problem is undertraining. The problem is high caregiver turnover. The problem is paying minimum wage. The problem is the eldercare industry. (I could go on, and so I will: The problem is undervaluing the elderly. The problem is fear of aging. The problem is fear of dying.) Some problems can be easily fixed and others can't. Whatever the problems, they are either ours to solve or, twenty or thirty or forty years from now, ours to live. I heard a nursing home director on a PBS documentary about eldercare say that if baby boomers want anything to be different for them, they better start taking action now. Those of us choosing facilities for our parents today, he said, will be living in places just like these unless we instigate change.

But pondering the kind of nursing home or assisting living residence you'd like to live in, should that be necessary, is admitting you will age and weaken and maybe get sick and surely die. No wonder no one wants to do it before they have to (or even then). Since I've been working at Maplewood, my husband and I have joked about our own potentially institutionalized future. Our nursing home will have batik bedspreads and posters of the Who. Tuesday morning the Tarot reader will come for a visit. Wednesday, after our Thai dinner, will be Bruce Springsteen Night. (We haven't figured out the exact activities yet.) Friday: Cherry Garcia ice cream socials with hash brownies. In craft class we will tie-dye men's undershirts. That's as far as we get, the jokes, because we're like everyone else. We don't want to talk, let along think, about this. We're healthy and active and in our prime, and we'll always be healthy and active and in our prime. We'll live forever. Or, like my great-grandmother, Old Oldie, we'll go to sleep one night in our own beds, healthy centenarians, and simply not wake up the next morning.

But Larry's comment, his shaky hands, the haunted look on his face, forces me to stop joking long enough to ask myself: If I do need help when I get older, if it becomes impossible for me to live independently, how do I want to live? Do I want to be cared for by an overworked, underpaid woman with so many chores to accomplish on her shift that she can barely spare a minute to talk to me? Do I want my "apartment" to look like a motel room? Do I want to eat dinner when the sun is still high in the sky? Of course not. Those aren't the important questions anyway. The important question is whether I—whether any of us—have the gumption, foresight, creativity, fearlessness, imagination, whatever it would take, to do something about eldercare before it's our turn. I am heartened, delighted, giddy after reading a story in the *New York Times* about a senior co-housing project in California. Instead of settling for lodgings in an assisted-living facility, a group of eighty-year-olds bought land together, hired an architect and a builder together, wrote rules and bylaws, and created a small, livable community with patios and garden space and quarters above the communal meeting room for a full-time nurse. Sign me up.

When I come in two days later for my next afternoon shift, I meet up with Eloise at the reception desk. This is unusual, as Eloise rarely ventures out of the neighborhood on her own. I wonder what's going on, but I don't have to wonder for too long. Eloise is in the throes of one of her "call Barbara now" rants. Every time Patty, the receptionist, gets off the phone or finishes checking in a visitor, Eloise is in there pitching.

"I want to talk to Barbara. Call Barbara. I need to talk to her." Her voice is edgy, not yet combative but going in that direction. Patty is giving her the line she and I and other RAs have given many times in the past, that Barbara is "still at work" and that Patty will call her later when Barbara gets home. Of course, if a resident really needed to speak to a family member, we would make the call. But Eloise is just going through her mid-afternoon anxiety moment, and it's our job to calm her and redirect her attention.

"We'll make that call later, Eloise," Patty says in her nicest, sweetest voice. Eloise looks for a moment like she has an inkling she is being played, but the moment passes. I take her hand and lead her back into the neighborhood. She shadows me as I put my things away, stands by me as I chat with the day-shift caregiver, follows me as I check the little refrigerator to see what we've got for snacks. I pat her hand, give her little hugs.

"What should I be doing?" she asks me. "Shouldn't I be doing something?" Today Eloise is just aware enough of her own confusion to be confused by it. When something is not right with Eloise, it touches me in a place, or to a depth, that I am not touched by the other residents. I tell Eloise I have a plan: suppose you take a little nap and then I wake you for the afternoon exercise session—Susan has already placed the chairs in a circle at the activity end of the neighborhood—and then we'll have dinner. She asks me a lot of questions about the exercise session, which at first I think is good because it is distracting her. But then I see that what's happening is she is talking herself into being worried about something else. Exactly when will the class start? And exactly where will it be? And who will wake her up? And what happens if she oversleeps? And where is her room anyway?

I answer each question, then talk her through it all several times again as we walk to her room. When she gets to the threshold, she stops. "I wish I would just die and get it over with," she says. She doesn't say this with any drama or force. In fact, in psychological circles you'd call this a "flat affect." I search for something to say, something that respects her intelligence, that does not deny how she feels but that offers some comfort.

This is very hard. Why *should* she want to live? I have never questioned this for myself. I have never had a suicidal moment. People just want to keep on living, don't they? There's this life force that can't be denied. People fight back from ghastly injuries; they survive horrible accidents, dreadful experiences. They cling to life; they claw at life. But Eloise. Why should Eloise want to live? I can't tell her she should want to live because of her grandchildren, who have made lives thousands of miles away and rarely see her. Or her daughters, one geographically distant, the other emotionally barricaded. I can't tell her about the cool morning air and the way the leaves on the oaks are turning crimson—the simple joys of being alive in the natural world—because she no longer experiences that world. She seldom ventures from this place. Her world is carpeted and beige and lit by fluorescents.

I am thinking all this at lightning speed, still holding Eloise's elbow, still poised, motionless at the threshold to her room. I run out my string, and then my mind goes blank. I don't know what to say. But I hear myself saying this: "You are what keeps me going, Eloise. I couldn't do this without you." Once I say it, I know it's true. It's not just how she comforted me on my first day back after dropping off my son at college. A day has not gone by since I started work here that Eloise has not taken my hand or patted my arm or stopped me in mid-stride and said thank you or said what a good girl I am or noted how hard I work. Each time she says it, even if she says it a half-dozen times in a single day, even if she catches me at my most harried, each time she says it I feel a sharp pang of pleasure. I am useful. I am wanted. I am making a difference in someone's life.

"Do you have any idea how important you are to me?" I ask her. She lifts her hand and smooths back the wisps of hair that have fallen across my face as she often does. That simple motion bypasses my brain and goes right to that place in my chest (exact location: two inches east and one inch south of my heart), that place that should be full of my mother, but isn't.

Eloise smooths back another strand of my hair. "You are so good to me," she says.

"You're easy to be good to."

She looks at me and laughs. It's a rueful, dismissive laugh, but there's also mischief in it, a sense of play. The Alzheimer's scuds away, a cloud on a windy day. "Me?" she says. "Why I can be a real bitch sometimes."

Later that evening, Eloise comes over, her face dark and troubled. She is back on Barbara. She wants Barbara to come and pick her up. She wants Barbara to come live here. She wants to call Barbara. I grab Eloise by her elegant bony shoulders, then cup my hand under her chin and make her look me in the eye. Barbara is not here right now, I tell her. But I'm here. Let's you and me get some tea and have a visit.

Eloise takes my hand and puts it to her cheek. "You are just what I want for a daughter," she tells me. If there are any sweeter words an older woman can say to a younger one, I've yet to hear them. I tell Eloise that I am no one's daughter anymore, that I lost my own mother. The truth is I never had her in the first place. Eloise strokes my hand. She has forgotten about Barbara for the moment, forgotten that she wants to go home. I say what I've wanted to say for months.

"Can I adopt you, Eloise? Will you be my adopted mother?" I mean it. Alzheimer's and all, I'll take Eloise. She smiles a huge smile.

"It's a deal," she says.

22

"I am losing my mind," a woman named Fran says in a documentary about Alzheimer's that I am rewatching at home on one of my days off. I have borrowed the videotape from my local chapter of the Alzheimer's Association, a little storefront staffed by volunteers so warm and cheerful you actually enjoy visiting the place. Illness can bring out the best in people. Fran, the woman in the videotape, is well put-together and early middle-aged. She's looking straight at the camera, forcing the viewing audience—that would be me—to make eye contact. It is hard to look a woman in the eye who says she's losing her mind.

But I have no choice. I am compelled by her tone, which is neither self-pitying nor resigned. It is in-your-face matter-of-fact. Fran is in the beginning stages of early-onset Alzheimer's, a disease with which she is far too familiar. An unlucky (and unusual) genetic configuration is embedded in the cambium of her family tree. Her mother had Alzheimer's. Her aunt had Alzheimer's. Her older siblings all have Alzheimer's. She knows what's coming.

"I am losing my mind," she says, looks down for a moment, then back up at the camera. "But the essence of a person is their heart, isn't it?" The documentarians let the question hang in the air. *Is the essence of a person head or heart?* It's not a warm-and-fuzzy New Agey question. It's a real question that goes to the core of our sense of what it means to be human: When we lose our mind (our memories, our coherent thoughts) do we lose our humanity? If we keep our "heart" (our emotions, our connectedness) do we remain, in essence, who we always were? When my mother got Alzheimer's, when I saw her and spent time with her, I would have answered that question, emphatically, one way. When you lose your mind, you lose your self, I would have said. Alzheimer's makes people into zombies, I would have said. The walking dead. Give me anything, but spare me this disease, I would have said.

But the time I've spent with the residents of Maplewood has eroded my certainty about this. When I see Jane laughing as she plays balloon ball or when I watch Old Frances eat ice cream as if it's a gift from the gods, when Eloise's eyes light up as I walk in the room, or when Hayes used to say something so stunningly perfect I swore he must have been reading from a very clever script, it is impossible to think of these people, disease and all, as anything less than fully human.

But sitting here watching this persistently grim documentary about a shattered family is not just a reminder for me of how most people think of Alzheimer's, of how I used to think of Alzheimer's, it is also a kind of reality check. It makes me consider the notion that, in looking to learn from this disease these past few months—and in finding so much that is positive—I may be in danger of overcompensating, of even romanticizing Alzheimer's.

How this is possible given some of the things I've seen—Ella spread-eagled on the floor of her bathroom, Rose wandering vacant-eyed through the halls—I don't know. But part of me has come to think of Alzheimer's, despite its obvious horrors, as a disease of freedom. It's not just memory that one loses. It is inhibition. It is pretense. The thin layer of civility that forces us healthy people to operate with equanimity even when we are tired or crabby or don't like someone or just want to be left alone—that's gone too. What remains is some unvarnished, unprotected self, maybe the self a person would have been had culture and society, gender and class, manners and mores not overlaid it. The buried self, the unlived self.

Of course, the human animal in the absence of all these civilizing conditions may not be all that pleasant. And family members accustomed to the pre-disease person who revealed only what he or she wanted to reveal, whose ego was fully in charge of the show, might very well find the new person difficult, distressing, even heartbreaking. I know I did. But there's one thing about the folks at Maplewood, about people with Alzheimer's in general: they are real, even the ones like Frances M. and Marianne, who are seriously deluded. They don't have ulterior motives. They don't manipulate. They don't play games. They just are.

I don't think I've overromanticized here. This is undoubtedly an alternate perspective that goes against the zombie stereotype, but it is not a through-rose-colored-glasses perspective (pun intentional). It is a way of looking past, or underneath, the disease to see the person. But there's another idea I've been mulling over, and it is far more controversial and perhaps crosses a line most people would be unable or unwilling to cross.

As I've been working at Maplewood and immersing myself in the quirky world of my residents, I've become a bit enchanted with the notion of Alzheimer's as Zen enlightenment. This Zen idea is not original with me. I got it not from a monk, not from an "alternative health care provider," but from the chair of the geriatrics department at Florida State University Medical School. I talked to him just before I started working at Maplewood. I was calling all around the country picking the brains of experts as I tried to get a handle on this disease. His name is Kenneth Brummel-Smith, and I remember that he took my call late on a Friday afternoon. He was leaving for a cross-country trip the next day and was in a rush to get out of his office, get home, and get packing. That is, he was in a rush until he started talking about a new way of looking at Alzheimer's. Impassioned people forget time.

"Now I know this sounds way out there," he told me, "but look at it this way: Alzheimer's is a detaching disease. It detaches people from their memories, their selves. We can look at that as tragic and awful, or we can change the frame." I didn't know where he was headed, but he had my attention. "Consider Zen," he said, "which is all about clearing your mind, detaching from your thoughts, grounding yourself in the moment." He paused, either to give me time to consider or for dramatic effect. "Well," he said finally, "that's Alzheimer's."

I didn't buy it then. It seemed absurdly Pollyannaish, delusional even, to characterize what everyone else seemed to think was a grim and tragic disease as the road to satori. But later, when I started to work at Maplewood, I saw how the disease forced people to live in the moment, to, as Ram Dass wrote, "be here now." And I understood what the doctor had been trying to tell me.

Later in the conversation, Brummel-Smith launched into a story about a monk who spent part of each day raking the sand in a Zen garden. It was a simple, repetitive act, and he did it the same way every day. He lost himself in it. "And we respect that," the doctor told me. "We see this man as enlightened." Those with Alzheimer's often perform simple, repetitive acts, he pointed out. But when we look at their repetitive acts, what we see is weirdness and disease. "Now just suppose we look at a person with Alzheimer's the same way we looked at the monk." He was speaking softly, and there was a kind of wonder in his voice you don't often hear in the voices of doctors.

I told him about a woman in my mother's care facility, a former university professor who spent hours folding and unfolding clothes. "But that's different," I insisted. "The monk was being mindful. This lady's actions were mind*less*." Brummel-Smith didn't say anything. He didn't need to. When I heard my words, I got it: The monk was mindfully trying to *achieve* mindlessness. He was working toward a state the woman folding clothes had already reached.

But it is hard to hold on to these wonderfully liberating views of Alzheimer's—as a disease of freedom, as a path to enlightenment—when you are changing adult diapers, or when the person with the disease is your mother, or when the media endlessly repeat wrenching and tragic tales. I think now I've reached some kind of equilibrium, a place between the two extremes. Hayes may not have been a crazy Zen monk, but neither was he a pitiable shell of a man. It is possible to look at Alzheimer's with a fresh point of view but without going overboard and making the disease into "a gift."

I've also been struggling to come to terms with something else as I've worked at Maplewood: my own fear, the fear that my mother's illness is in my genes. When I did all those interviews with experts, I spoke to a director at one of the country's top Alzheimer's research centers. Dr. Linda Boise had been working in the field for fourteen years, and while she had few illusions about the way Alzheimer's affected families, she also felt there was much life to be lived after diagnosis. Her husband, however, did not. *If I get Alzheimer's, just shoot me*, her husband had told her. I absolutely understood this. It was, in fact, how I felt at the time. During my mother's stay out West, I had made my husband promise, on more than one occasion, to stockpile enough pills so I could take my own life if I ever got Alzheimer's.

Now I'm not so sure. I think there are far worse ways to go, perhaps not for families but for the person with a disease. Would I rather spend my last six months gasping for breath with every exertion, bedridden with advanced coronary artery disease? Would I rather be hooked up to a morphine pump so I could manage the intolerable pain of end-stage cancer? Would I rather be on dialysis three times a week? These are perhaps not the questions a healthy, active (sane) person would ask herself, but they are, nevertheless, the questions this healthy, active (sane) person has asked herself. Spending months around people who are at the end of their lives cannot help but make you ponder the end of yours. And frankly, after months of such pondering, I now think I'd rather spend my waning days walking around clueless, holding a chocolate chip cookie in my hand, being hugged by big, pillowy women than lying in a hospital bed hooked up to IVs, alert, cognizant, with every memory intact.

That doesn't mean I've reached a détente with the disease, just that I'm not locked in hand-to-hand combat anymore. I don't want to get Alzheimer's as much as the next guy. I want the heroes in the white lab coats to come up with something amazing and definitive and *in time*. I monitor their progress through my Alzheimer's Google Alert. But I no longer panic every time I forget where I put my coffee cup, attentive to the little voice inside my head which asks, *Is this how it started with your mother?*

One day, I am alerted to a story about how genes are now thought to play a bigger part in late-onset Alzheimer's—bad news for me. The next day, that exercise and stimulating mental work can ward off the disease—good news for me. The more education you have, the longer you can stave off Alzheimer's. Yay! But, I read the very next day that the more education you have, the faster the disease progresses. I read that my lab-coated heroes have come up with a new compound that inhibits the proteins that lead to the inflammation that causes Alzheimer's— yes! In a test tube . . . Then there's the exciting new compound that relieves cognitive symptoms and reduces two kinds of brain lesions . . . in mice. It seems as if every week, scientists at some university posit a theory. Every week a biotech firm announces a new drug. Every month a clinic or hospital announces a new study. A person could go crazy following this news. Sometimes it's a relief to be at work, in the trenches with the disease, instead of sitting at a computer inundated by updates.

23

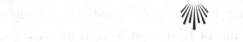

"So, have you heard about the new after-hours phone message they have here?" The woman asking the question, which is not actually a question but rather a setup for a joke, is a stand-up comedienne, the star attraction at Maplewood's first-ever Caregiver Appreciation Night. "Well, I called in the other night, and let me tell you how it goes," the comedienne says.

"Hello, you have reached Maplewood." She imitates the clipped, disembodied voice you often hear on prerecorded messages. *"Please press one if you want to talk to a staff member. . . . Please press two if you want to talk to a resident. . . . Please press three if you forgot who you want to talk to."* She pauses to wait for the laughter. It comes, but hesitantly, as if some people are deciding whether it's okay to laugh at stuff like this. *"Please press four if you forgot why you called."* More laughter, easier now. *"Please press five if you forgot who you are."* The comedienne has to raise her voice to be heard over the laughs. *"If you forgot how to use a telephone,"* she says, still imitating the recorded voice, *"just bang your head against the keypad."*

Now the entire room erupts in laughter. The event, orchestrated by Brooke, is taking place in the atrium at Maplewood. The comedienne, a woman named Leigh Ann Jasheway, has a national reputation in the small but feisty world of middle-aged female comics making fun of being middle-aged females. She tours, writes a humor column, and is the author of eight books, including *I'm Not Getting Older, I'm Getting Better at Denial*. Brooke snagged her for the event because Leigh Ann's mother-in-law is a resident at Maplewood.

"Hey," Leigh Ann says, when the laughter almost dies down. "Did you see the graffiti in the bathroom in neighborhood 1?" She cocks her head to one side and makes us wait a heartbeat for the next line. "It says: For a good time, call 9-1-1."

I laugh along with a roomful of my fellow RAs and fifty or so family members and try to imagine what "outsiders" would think of all this. *Laughing at Alzheimer's? A crowd of institutional caregivers and devastated family members guffawing at a tragic disease?* Are we all sick or something? The way most people would understand Leigh Ann's shtick is as gallows humor. The gallows, the big, bad, nasty thing out there—Alzheimer's, aging, illness, death, take your pick—is so big and bad and nasty, so devastating, that you find humor in it because you have to, because humor is what makes the unbearable bearable. There's truth to that view. There is an element of gallows humor, but that's not all that's going on here. I think we in this room are not a bunch of tortured souls laughing because, if we didn't, we'd put a collective gun to our collective head. We are, rather, an odd group of people who see in this Alzheimer's world life and light where others may see only darkness and despair. To us, Leigh Ann's humor is a natural part of a world that is itself full of humor—if a person chooses to see it that way.

The crowd is mostly middle-aged or—in the case of the old-before-their-time thirtysomething RAs—looks middle-aged. Maybe that's why the next joke gets the biggest laugh of the evening.

"I heard that twenty percent of women say their sex life is *better* after menopause," Leigh Ann says, looking out at us and nodding knowingly. "Of course that could just be the memory loss. Now I'm not saying these women forget how good sex used to be . . . I'm saying they forget where they live and end up having sex with neighbors." The crowd eats it up.

I look around the room and count more than two dozen RAs, most of whom are dressed in what used to be called "Sunday best"—skirts, dresses, even heels—many of whom are wearing makeup and none of whom have their hair scraped back in the usual and unfailingly unflattering workaday ponytails. It's the first time since Hayes's funeral that I've seen any of my coworkers out of uniform. They are sitting interspersed among the family members of the residents, just the families I would have imagined would be here, the ones who visit often, the ones who stop to talk to us in the neighborhoods, the ones who see us as vital to their mother's or father's care.

Brooke has spent some money on this event, either squeezing funds from Maplewood's operating budget or getting Corporate to ante up. There are platters of catered food. Nothing too fancy—deli meats, crudités, crackers, and cheese—but for minimum-wage slaves accustomed to eating Taco Time out of a bag on their way home from work, this is first-class chow. I give a fleeting and wistful thought to how else this money could have been spent: new uniform shirts, a few comfortable chairs out on the little patio we use at break, twenty-five-dollar Christmas bonus checks. I start to get angry, thinking about all the other things we need but don't have, until I look around again and see family members talking, shaking hands with and hugging RAs, until I see RAs nodding, beaming, and hugging back.

Jennie, Hayes's daughter, sees me from across the room and walks over with a big smile. It has been two months since Hayes died, but Jennie came tonight anyway. She tells me how thankful she is that we took such good care of her father. She tells me how much she misses visiting Maplewood, how much a part of her life this place became. Pam's daughter finds me and says how much she appreciates what I do for her mother. Addie's son waves from across the room. Jane's daughter gives me a thumbs-up. This event, whatever it cost, whatever it didn't buy for us, means something important to everyone here.

I'm struck—and not for the first time—by the inherent ironies of working here: Maplewood, an "institution," is providing consistently safer, kinder care than most residents could get at home. Family members know that. That's why they are here thanking us. The other major irony is that the residents' often empowering and enriching experience at Maplewood is being provided by a careworn and impoverished workforce.

After a half hour of eating and mingling and hugging—this is a roomful of huggers—Brooke calls for attention from the podium. A few family members want to say something. Up steps Duffy, a red-cheeked, jovial man in his mid-eighties whose wife of sixty-five years is a resident here in neighborhood 2. He visits her every day. He eats lunch with her every day. In the summer he brings her flowers from the garden every day. The staff loves him. Vernita, he says, referring to his wife, "is the most wonderful, most beautiful woman in the world." He says *is* not *was*. "And you all," he says with a slight catch in his throat, "are the finest caregivers this side of heaven." Then Pam's son stands up. "Sometimes we don't get a chance to say it. Sometimes we're too frazzled or you're too busy. But believe me, we see what you do every day, and we can't thank you enough."

For the next part of the program, Brooke asks all the RAs to line up by the side of the podium. She wants to read out our names, recognize our contributions, hand us certificates of appreciation. I see the other RAs set down their plates of food, stand up, brush off their skirts, and walk self-consciously to the front of the room. I watch a queue form. But I stay in my seat. All of a sudden, I am unsure of my status here. Am I considered a bonafide worker, a time-clock-punching employee worthy of being recognized and appreciated? Or does Brooke think of me a writer posing as an RA? I know how *I* feel about it: I work hard. I'm not pretending. But if my name is not on Brooke's list, I'll be left standing up there feeling foolish.

Brooke looks at the RAs forming a line to her right, then scans the audience. "Come on," she says. "We want all of you up here." Two more women get up to join the line. I'm still in my seat. On her next scan, Brooke sees me in the audience, smiles, and motions me with her head. I know it's okay now. I join the group.

She calls our names, one by one, and we walk to the podium to pick up our certificates along with a single long-stemmed red rose. Here comes Cathy, who gave me such a hard time early on but with whom I've reached a détente, and Lena, the talker, the chain-smoker, who regaled me with tales from her imperfect life. There's Anastasia, who almost turned me off to the job on my second day, and Inez, whose patience and equanimity saw me through rough times on swing shift. The audience claps hard for each of us. I wish Jasmine was here. She should get a rose too. She should hear people applaud for her.

When we're all back in our seats, Brooke says she has a special announcement to make. She will now present the first-ever

Employee of the Year Award. I have one monstrously egotistical—
but thankfully fast-fleeting—thought: Wouldn't it be great if *I*
were named Employee of the Year? Seeing as how five minutes
ago I wasn't even sure I would get a certificate, this is not just a
wildly inflated thought but a silly one as well. Anyway, I know
who really deserves this. I know who works hard and makes it
look easy, who is somehow quick and efficient yet also relaxed
and patient, simultaneously clear-eyed and compassionate, a
quiet force, a natural. She knows every resident and has worked
every neighborhood. She's the one you want on your shift. She's
the one you want backing you up. I can't imagine the award going to anyone other than my trainer, Calm Guam Frances.

When Brooke calls her name, Frances is the only one in the
room who is surprised. The family members turn to each other
and nod. The RAs stand and hoot. Frances walks to the podium
to get a bouquet and a hundred-dollar check. Her placid face is
only ever so slightly less placid, but I see she has tears in her
eyes.

Two days later I am back in neighborhood 3. This is probably
my last day. Okay, it *is* my last day. But I can't quite admit it. I
haven't signed up for any more hours. I am not on the December schedule at all. The truth is, my "fieldwork" is done, and I
must now begin to carve out time for thinking and writing. I
know that my family's patience is growing thin. There is no
question that my work at Maplewood has an impact on them.
When I work day shift, I'm out of the house before 6:00 a.m. I
don't see the kids, can't check to make sure they've remembered
their homework, their lunches. I leave my husband with the task
of getting them up, dressed, fed, and driven to school. When I
work swing, I'm gone all afternoon, not home when the kids
come back from school, not home to help with homework, to

cook dinner, or be part of the family during those few evening hours when we're all together. It's hard to imagine what a day-in, day-out schedule like this would do to a family, what it does to millions of families.

So, today, for reasons both personal and professional, will be my last day. Still I can't bring myself to tell Christine, who is in her crowded little office putting together the work schedule. I tell her instead that I'm not signing up for any December hours. She looks disappointed.

"You're still going to work here, aren't you?" she asks. I hedge.

"It's hard to say," I tell her. "I'm just not sure what I'll do after Thanksgiving."

"How would you like a permanent full-time job?" she asks. She's teasing, I think, but I am so pleased. I pass muster. It matters to me that Christine would hire me on. She's tough. She's been here longer than anyone else, working her way up from RA to Med Aide to her current position, low man on the administrative totem pole. She hears everything, every complaint, every piece of gossip. She's seen RAs come and go.

"We always need good people," she says. "You *know* you want to stay. You *know* it's in your blood." She's right. I smile. I can't think of anything to say.

I stride into the neighborhood determined to be supergirl today. I am going to be the best RA this side of Calm Guam Frances. I am going to do everything right, and I am going to do it all with grace. I'm on day shift today, which means more work but fewer behaviors. I get to it immediately, greeting Eloise, who is already awake, dressed, and seated at the table. Eloise will be the hardest part of leaving here.

I walk up to her, smiling, but she doesn't return the look. Her face is pinched and anxious.

"Have I done anything wrong?" she asks me before I have a chance to say hello. "I haven't done anything wrong, have I?" I tell her no, of course not, and good morning and would you like a cup of coffee.

"What have I done wrong?" she asks again. Nothing, not a thing, I tell her again, although I can see this is doing no good. I wonder where this comes from, this free-floating anxiety, these suspicions she has that she's done something wrong. And I wonder what her definition is of "something wrong." My guess is she means inappropriate behavior. Perhaps she is concerned that she might have said something or done something weird or embarrassing, which would be bad enough, but on top of that, she might be troubled by the fact that she can't remember doing it. Maybe there's a battle going on somewhere inside Eloise between her "liberated" Alzheimer's self, the new woman who is free of restraints and might do or say just about anything, and the old Eloise, the woman of social graces and impeccable manners. Or maybe I am trying to read too much into it. Understanding Eloise has become very important to me.

I know that nagging feeling that something is not quite right, but you can't remember what it might be. I'll wake up like that sometimes, not often, but sometimes. And maybe it will turn out to be a phone call I haven't returned or a meeting I missed, nothing big, but enough to create a dis-ease. I think many people with Alzheimer's live with that dis-ease every day.

"I'm just so much trouble," Eloise tells me, after I've reassured her yet again, hugged her, rubbed her back. "You must have so much else to do."

"No, I don't," I say, lying.

I took a picture of Eloise last week, and when I showed it to my husband, he was silent for a long moment.

"She looks a lot like your mother," he said. "I mean, what your mother would have looked like had she lived longer." I hadn't seen that. I studied the image of Eloise looking for what he saw. Maybe a little in the face, in that slightly gaunt boniness they both have. The pale papery skin. Is it really that simple: I am drawn to Eloise because she looks like my mother? I don't buy it. In fact, I think I am drawn to Eloise because she is so much *unlike* my mother. She is so much how I wish my mother would have been, not just at the end, but in the beginning and in the middle too: warm, responsive, loving.

Eloise isn't the only one out in the common area when I first arrive. The noc shift RA has already awakened and dressed Old Frances and Larry, part of a new plan to equalize the workload between the two shifts, noc having the fewest chores, day having the most. Brooke came up with this plan out of necessity. We now have more residents than ever, and day shift, always a little insane, was becoming absolutely unmanageable.

It used to be that when I came on day shift at 6:30, no one was awake or dressed except for Pam, and that was because she slept on the couch in the living room and never took off her clothes. I had to get everyone up, dressed, toileted, and at the breakfast table by the time the food cart arrived at 8:15. If I really, really hustled, and if no one gave me too much of a problem, I could maybe accomplish this when there were ten or eleven residents in the neighborhood. But now there are thirteen.

The population is up in all the neighborhoods. I wonder if it's just the ebb and flow of the place and the fact that for the past two months there hasn't been much ebb—no one has died since Hayes and Rose; no one has been transferred to another facility—but there has been flow. New people have arrived to fill vacant rooms. That's not surprising. There is no shortage of people being diagnosed with Alzheimer's out there. But then that was true back when Maplewood had empty rooms in every neighborhood.

I ask Brooke why she thinks Maplewood is close to capacity right now. This is a big feather in her cap, so of course she's delighted to talk about it. And being Brooke, she is generous and humble in her answer. She says it's because the right administrative team is finally in place and that together they deliver "excellent customer service." The customers to whom Brooke refers are not the residents but the family members footing the bill. The "team," I think, is mostly her. Brooke spends hours on the phone and in private meetings with family members. She is on call every night and all weekend, available to talk, troubleshoot, problem solve, intervene, mediate, mollify, whatever it takes to keep the customers satisfied. I don't think Brooke manipulates or goes for the quick fix. I think she sincerely—and almost always good-naturedly—tries to deal with everyone's issues and concerns. The job is so unrelentingly stressful that it would undo most people. It hasn't (yet) undone Brooke because she is very young and has a personality so sunny you need SPF15 to be in the same room with her. She was also a college athlete, so she's got that no-pain-no-gain thing going.

When I ask Susan, the activities coordinator, about the swell in Maplewood's population, she says it's because visitors—that is, prospective family member "customers" who tour the facility—see that this is a happy place with lots going on and so choose to put their relatives here. It's hard for anyone outside this world to imagine that a place like Maplewood could be a "happy" place, but it is.

One of the reasons this place is in my blood, one of the reasons I am finding it hard to admit that today is my last day, is that it *is* a happy place. The widely accepted notion that there is no quality of life for those with Alzheimer's is not widely—or for that matter narrowly—accepted here. Susan's programs are built on the idea that the residents are capable of enjoying life, even if they don't remember ten minutes later what it was they were enjoying. Her attitude is that these folks are not done living, and that attitude is at the heart of the vitality here. Maplewood *does* have a good vibe, and I'm sure that's attractive to family members in the throes of depression, grief, exhaustion, shell shock, whatever state they are in when they come here to visit, when they finally realize their mother or father needs more help than they can give.

Christine, hardheaded, practical Christine, has another explanation for the rise in population: Maplewood, unlike many other facilities in the area, is continuing to accept Medicaid patients. That means that residents without sufficient funds can live here, with the government picking up the tab. It also means that families who can afford to pay the bill right now know that if (or when) the money runs out, their relatives won't be kicked out of the place. Christine thinks, notwithstanding Brooke's administrative abilities or Susan's activity program, a family might choose Maplewood for this purely economic reason.

For the facility, the Medicaid-friendly policy is a tricky and challenging way to go. The government reimburses Maplewood fifteen hundred dollars a month for each resident on Medicaid. But Maplewood's least expensive monthly plan—the one designed for residents who can pretty much take care of themselves—is thirty-one hundred dollars. Brooke has said she has to be careful to watch the ratio of Medicaid to private-pay residents, so there must be some formula the corporation uses to make the economics work. Another way to make it work is to create as high a profit margin as possible for the private-pay residents, which means keeping down costs, which means bare-bones staffing, low wages for RAs, negligible health benefits for employees.

The RAs don't care why the place is filling up. What matters to us is that there are more people to care for, more chores to accomplish in the same amount of time, more work for the same pay. But Brooke's new plan to get noc shift to shoulder a bit of the morning burden is helping a little. And she has also managed to persuade Corporate to add one-half of one position for one shift—not an overwhelmingly magnanimous move, but any increase in staff, no matter how small, is good news. Now on day shift there is a full-time rather than a half-time Float, which means there is help serving noon meals and an increased chance that neighborhood RAs will actually get at least one of the two ten-minute breaks to which we're entitled.

And so this last morning feels, if not easy, then at least less harried. I wake the remaining residents, their faces and bodies familiar, their habits second nature to me now. It's difficult to remember, possible to imagine, that there was a time only a few months ago when I had trouble distinguishing between Old Frances and Addie. I don't see how I could have had a problem telling them apart. Except for the fact that they are both white-haired old ladies, they have almost nothing else in common, physically, emotionally, or otherwise. And back when I first started, I was flummoxed for days because there were two Franceses in the neighborhood, as if everything else about these two women did not adequately and definitively make them individuals, as if one might somehow confuse George Bush with George Clooney because they were both Georges. I was blind to obvious differences, oblivious to individual character in much the same way racists are when they insist they can't tell one Asian from another. Don't Chinese people look just like Japanese people who look just like Koreans? Well, yeah ... *if you never look. If you pay no attention.* That's how I was—how I think so many of us are—with old people. We simply don't see them.

Now I see. And at least I know *these* folks as individuals. I know the names of their daughters and sons and grandchildren. I know their moods and habits, their likes and dislikes. I know that Jane likes cornflakes every morning, that Marianne uses two packets of sugar in her coffee, that Eloise prefers sitting at the head of the big table, that Old Frances pulls her pant legs up over her knees and wants them that way. I have learned how things are done and to do them now without thinking. I remember when wheelchairs used to stump me, how I'd be down on my knees sweating when I had to swing the leg supports into place. I just couldn't figure out where things hooked and latched. I remember when I thought changing Pam's oxygen was so difficult that I called in the Med Aide to do it for me.

The morning zips by. An upbeat fellow named Byron comes in to lead the 10:00 a.m. exercise class. Then Rusty, a gorgeous Belgian Malinois shepherd, arrives with owner in tow and is admired and petted. The full-time Float rolls in the lunch cart. Everyone is served exactly what the meal schedule says he or she is supposed to be served. On my ten-minute break, I sit outside at the plastic picnic table in the covered area out by the garbage cans. It is a cold, gray day, typical for Oregon in late November. I sit protected from the thin drizzle listening to the sound of slick tires on the wet road. It occurs to me that I've watched two seasons go by sitting at this table.

In the afternoon, I polish Jane's nails, eat a piece of candy with Pam, chat with Marianne, play Legos with Larry, and give Eloise a shoulder massage in between doing three loads of laundry and toileting Addie and Old Frances. For my final act, the pièce de résistance of my last day, I cajole Millie, our most stubborn and recalcitrant resident, into the bathroom and give her a shower.

At 2:30, when the shift ends, I don't say good-bye to the residents. It would be confusing to some of them, meaningless to others. And too sad for me. Also, I know I'll be back. I'll come back some mid-morning to watch the show when Susan brings in the one-legged rooster or the potty-trained llama and the residents point and nudge each other and laugh. Or I'll come back mid-afternoon to sit on the couch between Pam and Jane while they watch *Singin' in the Rain*. One day I'll let Jim show me more of his baseball card collection. Another day I'll sit in Marianne's room with her and pretend it's her office. For Eloise, though, I have something else in mind. I have asked Barbara if I can take her mother out to lunch every so often. I want to be part of Eloise's life.

24

"You're back! You're back!" Patty, the receptionist, jumps up from her chair and runs out to greet me. We stand eye-to-eye thanks to the almost three-inch heels she is wearing. She gives me one of her signature full-body-contact hugs. I can't remember the last time anyone has been this happy to see me.

When I tell her that I'm here to visit, not to work, she starts to give me a hard time. Christine, hearing the commotion, comes out of her office and joins in. They're kidding, but they're not kidding. They really miss me. They really want me back. It's been three weeks since my last shift at Maplewood.

"I came to take Eloise to lunch," I tell them. I say this deadpan, but I know it is a startling statement. No one but relatives come to take people out of the building. That's the first surprise. The second is that Barbara, Eloise's daughter, would have granted me the necessary permission for this outing.

"Wow," says Christine. "I'm impressed." She touches her index finger to her tongue, then touches the finger to my forearm. "*Psssst*. You're hot, girl," she says. "How'd you manage that?"

It must seem like quite a feat, considering that it's doubtful anyone here has ever exchanged a friendly word with Barbara. The staff finds her difficult and unapproachable—which she is. She cares about Eloise and the treatment her mother gets at Maplewood, which is good and admirable and would normally make her a staff favorite. The problem is she expresses her concerns—which most of us would agree with—as sharp criticism. She walks in the door unhappy and walks out leaving everyone else worse for the encounter.

I'm not exactly sure why I am being permitted to take Eloise to lunch. It's not that I've been able to establish great rapport with Barbara, although I have certainly tried. Sometimes I think I understand Barbara and that after just one more conversation, just one more chance meeting in the grocery store we both frequent, I'll break through to whatever lies underneath that armor she wears. Other times, I think that what I imagine as understanding is really projection. Because I was angry and afraid when I visited my mother, I think Barbara is too. I think that her sharpness with others must be the way she copes with or hides her anxiety and fear. I can't imagine I'll ever know if this is true. But believing it to be true, choosing to see Barbara as scared rather than hostile means that I am better able to interact with her, that I take offense less.

When I first broached the subject of taking Eloise out to lunch, Barbara looked at me as if I'd suggested a fun outing at the endodontist. "Why would you want to do *that*?" She almost snapped at me. *Because Eloise needs love*, I wanted to say. *Because I need Eloise,* I wanted to say. "I think it would be nice for her," I said instead. "She loves to get dressed up, and this would be an excuse." Barbara opined that I wouldn't be able to handle Eloise outside of Maplewood. I decided not to be offended. I thought it was interesting that she doubted my abilities, given that I'd had sole responsibility for eleven people on my Maple-wood shifts. I told her I felt confident, but she shook her head no.

A week later, I suggested we all go out for lunch—Barbara, Eloise, and me. Again, she looked at me funny, but this time she said okay. I think she agreed because she might have been less than comfortable going out with Eloise alone, just as I had been when I took my mother out into the world. *Would she act weird in public? Would she pee in her pants? What would happen if I lost control of the situation?* I was always on high alert, never able to relax. Perhaps Barbara felt that way too.

Whether that was the reason or there was another, I don't know. But Barbara agreed to the lunch, and when we got to-gether at a Mexican restaurant, it went well. Eloise was mostly quiet. Her table manners were impeccable. How I think I won over Barbara that day was that I noticed Eloise squirming in her seat, suggested a trip to the bathroom, and negotiated the excursion pleasantly and efficiently. No fuss, no bother, no condescension, no I-am-taking-a-demented-lady-to-the-bathroom attitude. When I called Barbara a few days later to ask about tak-ing Eloise out alone, she said she'd permit it. She would call Patty and tell her it was okay.

And so here I am, dressed in a nice pair of slacks, my nine-year-old daughter waiting in the lobby, ready to take Eloise out for lunch. I've chosen the same restaurant that I took my parents to many years ago when they were out visiting. It's the kind of place one takes one's parents: not too fancy, but fancy enough; easily recognizable menu items; waitstaff who do not find it nec-essary to act like they're smarter than you are. Eloise looks lovely. She is wearing an ivory-colored silk blouse, accented by a gold brooch. She is wearing lipstick.

"How nice to see you," she says, greeting me in that sincere, well-mannered, but purposely vague way she has of greeting everyone. It's as if she's hedging her bets. The greeting is warm enough so that if she's supposed to know who you are, it works. But it's noncommittal enough so that if you happen to be a stranger, she isn't implying otherwise. Sometimes I think the Alzheimer's brain, at least at early- and mid-disease, is amazingly clever—all this mental maneuvering, this temporary relearning of what is instantly forgotten, these ways of using language to mask the decline of vocabulary. It's like the intact part of the brain is trying to outsmart the Alzheimer's part.

Eloise doesn't recognize me. But when I start talking about our having gone out to lunch with Barbara, when I put my arm around her and give her a hug, I can tell that something clicks. She doesn't know who I am, but she knows I am someone she knows.

She takes an immediate shine to my daughter, which makes everything easier. I've prepped Lizzie, told her that Eloise has a sickness that makes it difficult for her to remember. I've told her that Eloise might act a little strange, that she might say something odd. Lizzie is unfazed. She has accompanied me to Maplewood twice before, for a Halloween bash and the Hawaiian party, where she joined a group of slightly older girls who helped out by serving cake and punch. When I had asked her what she thought of the "grandmas and grandpas" at the party, she thought for moment, then said earnestly, explaining to me: "They just have their own way. It's like they're living at a different speed."

In the car driving to the restaurant, Eloise seems only mildly curious about where we're going. She looks out the window, hands folded in her lap, long, elegant fingers interlaced, but she doesn't seem to be tracking the moving landscape. Lizzie tries to start a conversation. "What's your favorite thing to have for lunch?" she asks from the backseat. I don't think Eloise hears the question. At any rate, she doesn't respond. I am too preoccupied to join in, engrossed as I am with conjuring the meaning and resonance of this lunch: The lunch my daughter, my mother, and I never had. The grandmother my daughter never knew. Healing the wounds of the motherless daughter. You name the Oprah issue, I'm thinking about it.

Eloise, of course, is unencumbered by the baggage I carry. She doesn't remember comforting me when I cried about my oldest child going to college. She doesn't remember that I've adopted her. She doesn't know how much she means to me. This is just a lunch. Right. We sit. We order. Lizzie butters a roll for Eloise, unasked. My daughter apparently has no trouble being in the moment, that's what childhood is all about, and Eloise has no trouble being in the moment, thanks to Alzheimer's. That just leaves me, in the middle, sitting here sorting through the past, imagining the future, oblivious to the present. I've got to get with the program.

The food comes, and I watch Eloise decide which piece of silverware to use. It takes her a while, but she chooses the right one. My daughter tucks into her plate of chicken strips, quietly amazed that I've allowed her to order deep-fried food.

"You're such a pretty little girl," Eloise says, between slow, careful bites. My daughter beams. Eloise says it again, a few minutes later, and then again. Lizzie shoots me a look, but she doesn't seem to mind the repetition. She is intent on the chicken strips, delighted to be at a restaurant where you aren't asked if you want to biggie-size anything, thrilled that I let her wear lip gloss for the occasion. We eat in companionable silence. Every once in a while, I reach over and pat Eloise's hand. Every once in a while Lizzie kicks me lightly under the table, and we smile at each other. Later, after we drop off Eloise at Maplewood and are driving home, Lizzie tells me that she's had a great time. She really likes Eloise, she says.

"That lady doesn't talk very much," Lizzie says. "But I understand why."

"Why?" I ask her. She looks annoyed. She hates having to spend time explaining the obvious to me.

"She's just a little shy being around a new family, Mom. She'll get used to us."

All of a sudden, Christmas is two weeks away. It's been close to a month since my last day at Maplewood. Susan calls me at home to remind me about the party next week, insisting that I come. Two days later, Brooke calls to remind me. I can hear Patty yelling in the background: "Tell her she better get her rear on over here." Brooke starts to repeat the message, but my laugh interrupts her.

"I guess you heard that, huh?" Brooke says.

When I arrive mid-afternoon a few days later, the normally deserted lobby is abuzz. Jim, one of the facility's two janitors (both of whom, conveniently and confusingly, are named Jim), is fiddling with a dead string of lights on the Christmas tree. Patty is futzing with holiday decorations on the end tables. Susan is rushing in and out of the lobby, carting in bakery boxes of sheet cakes from her car. In the corner, by a fake fireplace with painted ceramic logs pleasantly ablaze, stand two men and four women who look to be in their early twenties. The men wear morning coats and top hats. The women wear long velvet gowns with tight bodices. They are, I surmise, The Kings Carolers, the Elizabethan singing group Susan has lined up for entertainment.

The Carolers are in a tight huddle discussing the order of songs they'll sing today. One of them, a short woman in a dark green dress, says quietly to the others: "Don't let it throw you if we don't get much applause or if people don't seem to react. These people here all have Alzheimer's." The others nod solemnly.

Inside, sitting in chairs arranged around the perimeter of the atrium, are the residents. Fifty-six people live here now, which means every room is taken. There's even a waiting list. Maplewood has hit its stride, aided, no doubt, by an ad campaign on local TV. I've seen one of the commercials. It features Maplewood's favorite couple, Duffy and Vernita. Duffy is the apple-cheeked octogenarian husband who spends every day at Maplewood with his wife, Vernita, a big, smiling woman. The ad is simple and so unpretentious and homespun that you forget it's an ad. It's just Duffy and Vernita sitting together. He's holding her hand, looking at the camera through the chunky lenses of his old-guy glasses, talking about how he enjoys spending time with his wife at Maplewood. The message is simple and powerful: if this wonderful man who obviously dotes on his wife and wants the very best for her thinks this is a good place, it's got to be a good place. You couldn't ask for a better spokesman. I hope Duffy is getting a break on Vernita's monthly bill.

I see the two of them across the room, Vernita in her wheelchair, Duffy sitting so close his shoulder touches hers. There are dozens of family members here, the same dozens who always show up: Jane's daughter and son-in-law, Pam's son and two grandchildren, Frances M.'s daughter, Addie's son. And the same people are no-shows; the same residents sit alone. Maybe some family members are out of town. Maybe some don't live here at all. But I know there are those who just choose not to come.

This is another one of Susan's shining hours. Like the Hawaiian party she put on in the summer and the Halloween bash in the fall, it is a big, festive activity that involves residents, families, and staff, and gives a public face to the "life engagement" work she does every day. It's a time when music and food and activity animate this place and its people in a way that makes Alzheimer's almost bearable for even the saddest of families.

The middle school girls who volunteer to help at these events hand out paper plates of chocolate cake as The Kings Carolers begin their set. The singing is lovely—sweet, harmonic, pure, and joyous in that way Christmas carols and no other songs can be. I sit next to Brooke, who is looking gorgeous and visibly pregnant in a long scarlet dress. She has kept her pregnancy a secret for many months, something a six-foot-tall woman with expansive baby-growing room can do, something a woman like Brooke, with energy enough for three or four people, could pull off. She is now almost seven months pregnant and finally showing so much that she has to tell. She says she'll work until two weeks before her due date, then take a three-month leave and be back. The music washes over me as I watch the faces of the residents. Jane is smiling broadly. Eloise, unaccompanied by family, is nodding off. Old Frances is transfixed, her face tilted upward as if she thinks the music is coming from heaven, which it sounds as if it is.

I watch the RAs patrol the atrium, doing what I would be doing if I were on shift today. There are five of them working the room, one for each neighborhood and one Float, and they're easy to spot. In a room full of people in their holiday best— velvet and velour, reds, greens, and golds—they're the ones wearing the ugly purple-brown short-sleeved shirts. In a room full of people sitting, they are the ones in constant motion.

One woman in particular catches my eye. I can see that she's the one in charge of my neighborhood—yes, I still think of it as *my* neighborhood—and she's new. She is a big woman, her XXL Maplewood shirt tight across her gut, the polyester knit hugging three soft rolls of abdominal fat. Her hair is scraped back from her face in a greasy ponytail. I'm betting she is ten years younger than I am. I've never seen her before. I don't know her, but I bet I know her story, or some pretty close approximation thereof: lifelong minimum-wage slave. No money in the bank. Carts her dirty clothes to a strip mall laundromat every week.

I watch this woman as she walks slowly in front of the line of chairs set against the atrium wall. She nods and smiles at family members and stops at each resident. She squeezes a shoulder, pats a hand, ruffles hair, kisses a forehead, speaks a word or two. I think of Florence Nightingale walking among the wounded, not being able to do much but doing what she could. This new RA is soft and gentle, unharried. She is walking and smiling and touching, every move of her big ungainly body graceful and fluid. I am startled by how this work transforms her. She is beautiful.

I am an observer tonight. But because I once worked here, because I still feel the rhythm of this place in my bones, I see what others don't see. Vernita is getting antsy, and Duffy looks around for help. Before he gets himself up to find someone, an RA is there. I see that Caroline, wispy, red-haired Caroline, the former Rockette, is wiggling in her seat, a signal that she has to go to the bathroom. The new RA sees it too. Caroline isn't one of the residents in her neighborhood—*my* neighborhood—but the RA comes over anyway, helps her up, supports her by the elbow, and walks her to the bathroom. I see that Addie has fallen asleep in her wheelchair and is beginning to slump. Christine catches it a second after I do and goes over to lift Addie under the arms and reposition her.

The carolers launch into song after song, and after each one, there is thunderous applause. The young singers were concerned that the residents would not respond. They *assumed* the residents would not respond. But they were wrong. How little we all know about the experience of this disease. How surprised we are to learn life doesn't end when this disease begins. A half hour from now, when the carolers have left, very few residents will remember that these singers were ever here. That's only a tragedy if you choose to see it as a tragedy. You can choose not to. You can choose instead to focus on the faces of the residents as they listen. You can choose instead to see the pleasure they are experiencing right now, at this moment.

I close my eyes and try to achieve the now state that Alzheimer's grants to those from whom it robs so much else. I want to just listen to the music. In the brief intervals when I am not trying so hard to not think, I fall into the harmonies, and there is nothing else but the song inside my head.

The carolers are singing "Hark! the Herald Angels Sing" in four-part harmony, and it could make a believer out of anyone. I take deep, even breaths and listen, and then, all of a sudden, unbidden, comes a memory, a scene so sharply etched that I cannot believe this is the first time it has surfaced.

It is Christmastime eight years ago. I have come to see my mother, another in a long line of dutiful, depressing visits. Today, although it's cold and gray and threatening to rain, I take her out for a walk anyway. I'll do most anything to avoid just sitting with her. I'll do most anything to get out of the place she lives in. On my way over, a twenty-minute, crosstown drive, I always let myself cry for a few minutes. Then I crank up the radio and listen to bad rock 'n' roll, the kind seventeen-year-old guys in Camaros listen to. Then I give myself a pep talk: *You gotta do this. It won't be so bad. You owe it to her.* Still, the moment I walk in the door and see seven blank-eyed women, one of whom is my mother, sitting in the beige living room on a vinyl-covered couch with the Wal-Mart art on the walls, I want to get out.

So I bundle up my mother and take her for a walk through the quiet residential streets that surround her facility. It's drizzling, and she is talking nonstop, repeating the same phrase over and over again, as she often does. A few minutes before, at the beginning of our walk, I had seen a puddle on the sidewalk up ahead and had told her, "Be careful where you step." Since then, that's all she is saying: "Careful where you step, careful where you step, careful where you step, careful where you step." I can't get her to stop. It is driving me crazy.

Out of desperation, to drown her out, really, I start to sing "Rudolph the Red-Nosed Reindeer." I sing loud enough so I can no longer hear her, and so it takes a minute, a verse, maybe, for it to sink in that she's no longer talking. She's singing. Her speaking vocabulary has shrunk to a few dozen words, but she is singing along, remembering all the words to the song.

We go from "Rudolph" to "Frosty" to "Deck the Halls," without her missing a verse. Neither of us could ever carry a tune—my father always used to say I carried a tune on my back, and my mother was even more atonal than I am—and so we had both always been shy about singing aloud. But there we were, walking step by hesitant step, the sky blackening, the drizzle turning to rain, our sneakers soaked, our voices loud and off-key, and not giving a damn.

Epilogue

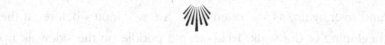

Nine months after I put my mother on a plane back to New York, my father called to tell me she was dead. That's one thing about my family: we don't mince words. No one uses phrases like *passed away*, or *passed on*. "Mom is dead," he said, without preamble. "She died this morning." He was calling mid-afternoon the day after Christmas. He didn't say, and I didn't want to ask, *how* she died. People will say someone "died of Alzheimer's," but Alzheimer's doesn't kill the way heart disease does, or cancer. I suppose, if a person somehow managed to stay alive long enough with the disease, theoretically neurological function could be so impaired that the brain could forget how to send signals to keep the heart beating or the lungs bellowing, and so a person could, in fact, die of Alzheimer's. But I can't imagine this actually happens.

We talked for a while on the phone, my father and I, both of us spouting the platitudes people spout in such circumstances, some of which are even true, like *It was good you were able to spend so much time with her*, and some of which are wishful thinking, like *She lived a good life*. Mostly he talked about funeral arrangements and burial plots while I half-listened. When we hung up, I called my brother. I had to know the details. I had to know how her story ended.

Her death was no surprise. I knew when she had gone back East that she didn't have much longer to live. Besides, I don't know if I'd thought of her as really alive the entire time she was out West with me. I didn't know then what I learned later at Maplewood—that people with Alzheimer's are still very much people—and so to me my mother, my "real" mother, had died a long time ago. This woman in the care facility, the one I forced myself to visit several times a week, was someone else.

But in the nine months since I'd last seen her, an odd thing had happened. I had replaced the disturbing image of that blank-eyed stranger with a picture of my mother as she was long before the disease, my mother with her curly coppery hair and lipsticked smile, my mother taking apart and repairing a table lamp, my mother grouting tile, my mother antiquing the dining room hutch, my mother in her little black dress with the plunging neckline, my beautiful, competent, talented mother, the mother of my childhood. It was this resurrected woman I somehow had to imagine dying, and I couldn't do it without the details. I needed to play the scene in my head, like a movie.

My mother, it turned out, choked on her breakfast. She died aspirating a piece of whole wheat toast. It didn't sound pleasant—so few ways of dying do—but it did sound fitting. Live by the sword, die by the sword. My mother, the dieter; my mother, the gourmet cook. My mother and her seven-decade love-hate affair with food. It made sense that a piece of toast did her in.

I didn't cry until much later.

———

It's been more than a year since I worked at Maplewood, but I still drive out there every so often. Things are different. A year is a long time in the life of an RA, most of whom don't last more than a few months at any one place. No one who worked shifts back when I worked is there any more. Lena and Cathy quit long ago, and no one knows where they are now. I have heard through the grapevine that Jasmine, who left while I was at Maplewood, is still taking classes at a community college while working part-time. I've heard she works swing at an Alzheimer's facility in another city. Calm Guam Frances, the best of us and the last to go, moved out of state a few months ago to start nursing school. I envy whoever is on the receiving end of her care.

There have been big changes in the administrative staff, too. Susan, ever optimistic, perennially perky Susan, quit to take full-time care of her stepfather, who was recently diagnosed with Alzheimer's. Christine, the care coordinator, quit to go back to school. She supports herself working noc-shift at the assisted living facility on Maplewood's aging-in-place campus. Brooke had a big, healthy boy and never came back from maternity leave. Only Patty of the old crew still works at Maplewood. She's now an assistant administrator.

A year is an even longer time in the life of a sick older person. Pam, whose oxygen tank I changed, and whose panic attacks I quelled, died of respiratory failure. Millie, the one I sweet-talked into a shower on my last day at Maplewood, broke her hip and never made it out of rehab. Old Frances, put on hospice for the eighth time last fall, finally succumbed, quietly, in bed, at age ninety-nine. Marianne is still alive, but she has declined dramatically. The most educated, erudite, and articulate of residents, she no longer speaks. She rarely wants to leave her room these days, and when she does, she moves slowly, with the aid of a walker.

But wheelchair-bound Addie, with her huge blue-gray eyes

and her devoted son who visits every afternoon, is still around. And half-pint Jane, the Energizer Bunny of the neighborhood, still takes constitutionals around the facility every day. When I visited a month ago, she remembered me.

Then there is Eloise. Walking in the neighborhood one day on the arm of an RA, she heard a sudden pop and was in immediate and significant pain. X-rays at the hospital revealed fractures in her pubic bone, thigh bone, and sacrum. I imagine her bones look like Swiss cheese. She was in the hospital and then in rehab for a long, long time, during which she lost thirty pounds and most of her mobility. Miraculously, she is back at Maplewood, where she has graduated from sitting in a wheelchair to using a walker. I am headed out there right now to see her.

Acknowledgments

I owe not only this book but a new way of thinking about age, illness, and death to the residents of Maplewood. What they taught me about patience and love, about character, and about what remains when it looks as if nothing is left, will stay with me forever. I owe an equally big debt to their relatives for allowing me into their lives at such a vulnerable and troubled time, for talking freely and honestly, and for giving me permission to explore their stories. I thank especially Janet Broadsword, Bill McLeary, Kevin McCarthy, Joby Patterson, Darlene Kennedy, Duffy Hamren, and Bev and Cal Foster.

I thank Maplewood's administrators, from Tricia Wagner and Jessica Feder, my early guides, to the irrepressible Brooke Cottle, my boss, for their extraordinary cooperation and openness. Without their support, there would be no book. I thank Christine Berra for giving me a schedule I could live with and believing I could do the job. I thank Susan Stuart Clark for showing me that life inside an Alzheimer's facility could be rich and rewarding, and Patty Neuman, for showing me it could be fun. I thank my overworked, underpaid coworkers—*and so should you all!*—for the amazing job they do every day: Jasmine Espenscheid, Inez Lowrie, Tiffany Cavin, Sandy Wahlbeck, Cynthia Camacho, and especially (Saint) Frances Chiguina.

Of all the many books and articles I read about Alzheimer's during the course of my research, I am most greatly and gratefully indebted to the work of Thomas Kitwood (*Dementia*

Reconsidered), James Hillman (especially *The Force of Character*), and Naomi Feil (especially *The Validation Breakthrough*). I thank Dan Reece; Liz von Wellsheim; Ron Stock, M.D.; Kenneth Brummel-Smith, M.D.; Linda Boise; Donna Peterson; and Debra Cherry for their insights about this disease and the care of those who suffer from it.

I thank Drex Heikes, former executive editor of the Sunday *Los Angeles Times Magazine*, for believing in *Dancing with Rose* when it was just an idea offered across the table at Allan Bros. Beanery one Saturday morning. The story I wrote for that magazine started me down this road, and it was Drex who made it happen. I thank interviewer extraordinaire Barry Kibrick of *Between the Lines* for his early and enthusiastic support.

I thank those who supported me and cheered me on: Perrie Patterson, Sabena Stark, Mariana Landazuri, Deborah Emin, Gail Miller, Sylvia Weisshaupt, Ami Simms, and the ghost of my incomparable Nanny, Dorothy Falk. I thank my friend, fitness buddy, and fellow shoe-aholic Lizzie Reis, who delivered thrice-weekly pep talks along the Amazon Trail and took time from her own important work to read and comment on mine.

I thank—and sing the praises of—my incredible team at Viking for their powerful combination of professionalism and passion: Molly Stern, my smart, savvy, and abundantly talented editor; Alessandra Lusardi, a sharp-eyed and gifted editor herself; Kate Griggs, Carla Bolte, Laura Tisdel, and Juliann Barbato (I've respected copyeditors before, but I've never *loved* one as I loved Juli). I thank my agent David Black, he of the hard head, soft heart, and smart mouth. I feel privileged to be represented by him and to count him as a friend.

And finally, and most especially, I thank Tom Hager, first reader, best editor, partner in life and literature.